Microdosing

For Health, Healing,
and Enhanced
Performance

Also by James Fadiman, PhD, and Jordan Gruber, JD

Your Symphony of Selves

Microdosing

For Health, Healing, and Enhanced Performance

* * *

**James Fadiman, PhD
and Jordan Gruber, JD
and hundreds of others**

ST. MARTIN'S
ESSENTIALS
NEW YORK

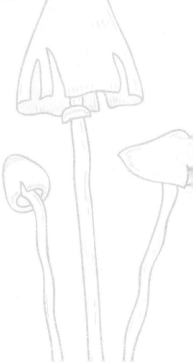

First published in the United States by St. Martin's Essentials, an imprint of St. Martin's Publishing Group

MICRODOSING FOR HEALTH, HEALING, AND ENHANCED PERFORMANCE. Copyright © 2025 by James Fadiman and Jordan Gruber. All rights reserved. Printed in the United States of America. For information, address St. Martin's Publishing Group, 120 Broadway, New York, NY 10271.

www.stmartins.com

Title page illustration by Shutterstock

The Library of Congress Cataloging-in-Publication Data is available upon request.

ISBN 978-1-250-35558-4 (hardcover)
ISBN 978-1-250-35559-1 (ebook)

Our books may be purchased in bulk for promotional, educational, or business use. Please contact your local bookseller or the Macmillan Corporate and Premium Sales Department at 1-800-221-7945, extension 5442, or by email at MacmillanSpecialMarkets@macmillan.com.

First Edition: 2025

10 9 8 7 6 5 4 3 2 1

To our families, friends, and
beloved animal companions

Disclaimers

Advice Not Provided: The information in this book, while accurate, complete, and up-to-date to the best of our knowledge, is presented for adult educational purposes only. As neither the authors nor the publisher are licensed medical or mental healthcare professionals, nothing in this book is meant to be taken as medical, mental health, spiritual, financial, business, or legal advice. The authors and publisher are not responsible for any negative consequences or damages that may arise from the use or misuse of any information provided, and assume no liability for unwise or unsafe actions taken by readers of this book.

Consult with Your Medical or Healthcare Giver: Please consult with a psychedelics-informed physician, healthcare provider, therapist, or pharmacist before engaging in any course of microdosing or *making any changes whatsoever* to your existing health and medication regimen, especially as to tapering off medications, or if you have any personal or family history of contraindicated medical or physical conditions, as described in the book.

Sourcing of Psychedelics: It is still illegal in many places to use or even possess psychedelics. The information found in this book is not intended to encourage or support illegal behavior, rather it is meant only to report on our understanding of results that have been experienced by people who have chosen to microdose. We do not and never will assist in the sourcing of psychedelics. This book does not provide legal advice regarding the use or possession of psychedelics.

Harm Reduction: If you mistakenly take a large dose of a psychedelic or otherwise need real-time support during a psychedelic experience, call or text 62-FIRESIDE in the US to reach the Fireside Project, or visit TripSit.me or ICEERS.org online and request phone support. The SHINE Collective at ShineSupport.org also provides support for those previously harmed by psychedelics. For questions about interactions between microdoses and medicines, see the appendix or MicrodosingInstitute.com. If at any point you feel substantially unwell or uncomfortable with any aspect of taking microdoses—stop. Never give someone a psychedelic of any kind or dose without their full consent. Finally, be extra cautious "microdosing" chocolate bars, gummies, or other candy, which can contain a wide mixture of substances, including synthetic analogues of psychedelics, and can be very dangerous. See the warning about the use of the word "microdose" and the US FDA Diamond Shruumz recall on page 12.

Third-Party Resources: Any third-party resources mentioned are provided solely for your convenience. The authors and publisher do not endorse or guarantee the services provided by any of these resources. Investigate on your own and use common sense.

Indigenous Acknowledgment: This book was conceived, written, and edited primarily on Ohlone land. We recognize that many traditional native and indigenous peoples have used plant medicines, including psychedelics, sometimes in ways that resemble modern microdosing. We intend to acknowledge and appreciate, rather than unconsciously or wrongfully appropriate, their contributions.

Contents

Preface   *xvii*

1. Overview   1

What You Will Find in This Book   1

Qualifications   4

Meaning of Microdosing   8

Safety   9

Why Microdose   12

Physical, Mental, and Spiritual Effects   13

Popularity   15

Concerns and Controversies   16

How Much Is a Microdose?   18

"Sub-Perceptual"   18

Reasons for Some People Not to Microdose   20

Value of Hesitation   22

Legality   23

Finding Substances   24

What Doctors, Therapists, Coaches, and Other
   Professionals Need to Know   24
Making Best Use of This Book   25

2. Basics   **27**

Substances Used for Microdosing   28
Other Substances   30
LSD   31
Psilocybin "Magic" Mushrooms   33
Illegal/Legal   35
LSD and Psilocybin Differences   37
How Microdoses Are Taken (and What With)   38
Dosage Ranges for Different Substances   44
Protocols: Keeping to a Schedule and
   Taking Breaks   58
Contraindications, Safety Concerns, and Other Cautions   64
Best Practices, Guidance, and Outside Assistance   72
Preliminaries: Introduction to Health Conditions and
   Symptoms Benefited   81

3. Enhanced Abilities, Wellness, and Flow   **86**

Cognitive Enhancement   87
Creativity Enhanced (Art)   88
Creativity Enhanced (Writing)   89
Focus   89
Food Choices   90
Grades and Academics   91
Happy (Truly)   92
Language Learning   94
Longevity   96
Math and Coding   97
Music (Creating and Performing)   98
Sexual Enhancement   98

Sleep Quality 99

Social Microdoses 100

Sports and Athletics 102

Vision Improvement 105

Work Quality Improvement 107

4. Current Findings of Special Interest 108

ADHD (Attention Deficit/Hyperactivity Disorder) 109

Depression 121

Long COVID 132

Microdosing Along With and Tapering Off Medications 137

Pain 139

Women's Health 144

5. Health Conditions Positively Affected 157

Introduction 157

Anorexia: A Case Study 159

Anxiety 162

Asthma Relief 164

Autism (Asperger's/High-Functioning) 166

Autism (Severe) and Children 169

Binge Eating 171

Bipolar Disorder 172

Body Weight 174

Cannabis Reduction or Quitting 175

Cerebral Palsy: A Case Study 176

Cluster Headaches 179

Color Blindness (Red-Green) 180

Common Cold 181

Dizziness (Perpetual): A Case Study 182

Eczema 183

Ehlers-Danlos Syndrome and an Accident: A Case Study 184

Epilepsy 188

Headaches (Migraine)   189

Inflammatory Bowel Disease (IBD)   190

Libido Lacking   191

Lupus: A Case Study   192

Lyme Disease (Persistent Lyme Disease Syndrome)   193

Multiple Sclerosis (MS): A Case Study   197

Palliative Care   200

Pornography Addiction   201

Post-Traumatic Stress Disorder (PTSD)   203

Premenstrual Dysphoric Disorder (PMDD)   206

Premenstrual Syndrome (PMS)   211

Schizophrenia   212

Sleep   214

Stroke   216

Stuttering   219

Traumatic Brain Injury (TBI)   221

Varicella-Zoster Virus (Shingles)   224

6. Science and History   **227**

Research Rising   227

Microdose.me Survey Results   229

Contemporary Observational Science   231

Citizen Science   237

Placebo Effect   238

Expectancy   241

Neuroplasticity, Neurogenesis, and the Default
    Mode Network   244

Inflammation   256

Potential Heart Damage Concerns   260

Homeopathy and Microdosing   262

Synthesized Psilocybin vs. Psychedelic Mushroom Extract   263

Indigenous Use   265

First Use of the Term "Microdosing" 270

Beginning of Modern Microdosing 272

7. Conclusions 275

What's Left Out 275

Some Additional Considerations 277

Predictions 278

Jim's Final Reflections 283

Jordan's Final Reflections 284

Acknowledgments 291

Appendix 299

Notes 303

References 313

Index 333

About the Authors 347

Microdosing

For Health, Healing, and Enhanced Performance

Preface

I've been investigating psychedelics, professionally and personally, since the early 1960s. Until fifteen years ago, I knew nothing about very small doses, nor did anyone else in my world. However, I've focused on little else since then, discovering, reviewing, and sharing the extraordinary results that people have reported after taking a tenth or less of a full-on psychedelic trip dose. During all those other decades I was fixated on transcendent doses (not concert, not recreational, not therapeutic, not even problem-solving). As I reflect on what I know now, I am filled with wonder and chagrin as well as gratitude and humility.

I was introduced to psychedelics one night at a sidewalk café in Paris in 1961, when my favorite professor, Richard Alpert (later Ram Dass), put a pill into my hand and said, "The greatest thing in the world has happened to me, and I want to share it with you." A few months later, no longer in Paris, I was a draft-dodging psychology graduate student at Stanford University. Apart from my academics, I worked off campus with a private clinic that was pioneering psychedelic psychotherapy. There, I took a high dose of LSD in a safe, guided environment and had a belief-shattering awakening, becoming aware of the interconnectedness of all things. That realization and its aftermath has shaped the rest of my life.

These days, there is an ever-expanding number of books by people recounting how all those astounding, amazing, fantastic trips changed their lives.

This is not one of those.

It is, instead, about how many thousands of people all over the world have improved their health and their capacities without the razzle-dazzle, heaven-opening, reality-expanding experiences that made the sixties such an optimistic, culture-changing decade.

While I've had some of those experiences, their main aftereffect was my becoming ever closer to nature and not overly attached to whatever I was doing. From the outside, my life looks remarkably normal. I've been married for sixty years; I have two daughters, both teachers; I've taught in three universities, owned three houses, drive a Prius (my third), and share our home with two small rescue dogs. I've edited and written a lot of books and articles, and in recent years, been in many videos and podcasts.

I was introduced to the idea of taking microdoses during a lunch at a Greek restaurant in Santa Cruz, California. Since then, I've been involved pretty much full-time with compiling their effects. I soon discovered for myself that itty-bitty amounts of LSD or psilocybin didn't take you on a small trip or even a short one; instead, taken over time, they produced a spectrum of beneficial effects that do not even remotely resemble the explosive revelations of higher doses. I also learned that almost no one in the psychedelic subcultures—including underground chemists, guides, psychonauts, and even the few aboveground researchers, scientists, and explorers—knew anything about these low-dose effects either.

This book is a compilation of more than a decade of reports from thousands of individuals from dozens of countries about a wide variety of health conditions as well as scientific investigations of these improvements. Jordan and I teamed up to write the book because we knew that sharing so much unknown, unpublished, and potentially paradigm-shifting information might alleviate an amazing amount of unnecessary suffering, and allow people to better develop their own skills and capacities. It could aid in stimulating research, almost all of which has been undertaken as scientists began to hear of the sorts of reports that fill this book. It could also encourage investment in making these substances more widely available, and help do away with the legal barriers that prevent people from improving their lives—regulations that never made sense in the first place.

Even as we complete this book, researchers, coaches, and individuals around the world are birthing a new field that works with microdoses to affect multiple physical and mental systems to enhance both medical treatments and healthy capacities.

—Jim Fadiman, May 17, 2024

PS: As you read along, you'll see that we're asking you in quite a few places to send in anonymous reports of your own experiences at Micro dosingBook.com. In this way, you can share what you know with others and encourage greater understanding, wherever you are along this path.

[1]

Overview

What You Will Find in This Book

You will find what you need to know about microdosing, from the most basic practical and safety concerns to specific protocols for special conditions. We bring you effective ways of doing things by presenting the best available information we know of, collected from many sources. Current research on microdosing is highlighted, along with its history and controversies. We focus, primarily, on the many reports from people who have shared their microdosing experiences to help others.

We have reviewed thousands of people's experiences, and all the research studies to date. Some of the information covered in chapters 3, 4, and 5—"Enhanced Abilities, Wellness, and Flow," "Current Findings of Special Interest," and "Health Conditions Positively Affected"—has not been reported elsewhere. Despite our best efforts, some of what's put forward in these pages *may prove to be partially or fully incorrect*. More complete information and new pathways of discovery will continue to emerge.

The effects of microdosing on many of the conditions we cover—like shingles or Lyme disease—are not yet formally researched. Any book about healing practices is a snapshot of what is currently known, filtered through the existing culture's set of beliefs and assumptions. This book is no different. Check for other sources if you can before exploring microdosing for yourself or recommending it to others.

Mainly using a Question & Answer (Q&A) format, we'll be covering the following areas:

- **Overview:** Starting with our qualifications, definitions, and safety concerns, we consider why people microdose and why it has become popular, the value of hesitation, and some legal and sourcing issues.
- **Basics:** We describe different microdosing substances—how they're taken and how much to take, what they're taken with, and how often to take them—as well as contraindications, safety concerns, and best practices.
- **Enhanced Abilities, Wellness, and Flow:** Here we look at things microdosing can help make better, from academics to work quality, spanning everything from music and sports to chess, coding, and sex.
- **Current Findings of Special Interest:** We take a close look at six areas where microdosing can possibly make a big difference—ADHD, depression, tapering off medications, long COVID, pain, and women's health.
- **Health Conditions Positively Affected:** We report on more than thirty physical and mental medical conditions that have seen healing and improvement, from anorexia, anxiety, and asthma relief to stroke, traumatic brain injury, and the varicella-zoster virus (shingles).
- **Science and History:** We look at some of the science and history relevant to modern microdosing, from neuroplasticity, inflammation, and the placebo effect to citizen science, ob-

servational science, and heart valve safety concerns. Included
is the story of how modern microdosing came into being, and
the relationship of modern practices to indigenous ones.

- **Conclusions:** What directions we look forward to and a few
  we worry about.

What you *won't* find in this book is specific information about
sourcing psychedelics, or recommendations for microdosing coaches or
courses. You're necessarily on your own for both of these, so be prudent
and make good choices. While this book contains a good deal of information, it isn't (and couldn't be) fully comprehensive. Microdosing
results keep coming in from all over the world, from personal reports,
surveys, and media interviews to academic and commercial research.

So if you don't see what you're interested in—a physical or mental condition that you or someone you care for is suffering from—
please don't lose heart. More information flows in daily about conditions
treated, abilities enhanced, substances being used, special protocols,
and so on.

Also, to the degree microdosing apparently—

- accelerates the placebo process
- releases natural healing factors that return us to a healthier
  equilibrium
- decreases inflammation
- increases neuroplasticity

—it is *potentially* helpful for any physical or mental condition. Feeling
better and more balanced generally benefits nearly any kind of physical
or mental concern, and supports enhanced abilities, wellness, and flow.
Like better sleep or a healthy diet, microdosing gives the body a leg up
toward healthier functioning.

Finally, if you are interested in a specific health condition or a potentially improved ability not mentioned here, we encourage you to go online and look for yourself. You can do a general online search or go to Reddit's r/microdosing subreddit. If you decide to do your own research, including self-study, please contact us through the MicrodosingBook .com website and let us know what you find; that's how most of what you're reading came to be included in this book.

Qualifications

What qualifies you to write this book?

Jim Fadiman's credentials include a BA from Harvard and a PhD in psychology from Stanford, as well as writing a variety of books (textbooks, professional books, and popular books, plus a novel), teaching in three universities, and holding many other jobs. He had just finished his dissertation on the effectiveness of LSD therapy when the government proclaimed how scary and dangerous psychedelics were before soon making them illegal. The chairman of his dissertation committee warned him that his LSD dissertation would be an academic career killer. (As Jim likes to say, "Fortunately, he was right.")

As he learned and shared about microdosing, Jim's research activities catalyzed what can be called "modern microdosing." Whether or not he was the first active researcher to personally microdose, he *was* the first psychedelics-trained psychologist to seriously explore its possibilities. He was also the first person to:

- describe microdosing's effects
- develop a "protocol" (a schedule) to maximize safe and beneficial results
- determine average safe and effective dose ranges for different psychedelics
- attract academic, clinical, and public attention for microdosing, now an expanding worldwide phenomenon[1]

During the forty years that legal psychedelic research was suppressed, underground chemists supplied—and millions of people took—high doses of psychedelics, often LSD.

Like nearly everyone else who remained interested in psychedelics during this period, Jim didn't have the faintest awareness of microdosing. For the most part, he focused on doses of LSD or psilocybin large enough to induce transcendent revelations. Jim notes that:

> Given my history, it is more than a little ironic that for the last fifteen years I have been exclusively exploring the tiniest of doses—ones that provide no classic psychedelic effects, no visual distortions, no instant therapeutic miracles, no life-changing spiritual epiphanies, and no deep real-time awareness of the interconnectivity of all things. Specifically, I have been collecting and organizing thousands of microdosing reports.
>
> I've been dubbed the "Father of Modern Microdosing" mostly because of my ongoing sharing of stories on podcasts, at conferences, in the popular press, and even in peer-reviewed journals. When I ask people to write me their story, I let them know that I will be passing it on so that others can benefit. These stories pave the way forward, enabling us to collectively become wiser and more adept at microdosing.

One of the people Jim shared his stories with was Jordan Gruber,* a former attorney, writer, and editor with a long-time interest in psychology, psychedelics, and human potential. Shortly after Jordan moved to California, he met Jim at a psychedelics conference, and living a

---

*Jordan has a BA in philosophy and a master's in public policy analysis and administration from Binghamton University, and a law degree from the University of Virginia. After briefly practicing law, he founded the Enlightenment.Com website.

mile and a half apart, they soon became close personal friends. After Jordan helped Jim with a small part of *The Psychedelic Explorer's Guide* around 2010, they worked together from 2015 to 2020 to coauthor *Your Symphony of Selves: Discover and Understand More of Who We Are* (Park Street Press) on the idea of "healthy multiplicity."

They have teamed up again to write *Microdosing for Health, Healing, and Enhanced Performance.* They agreed that this book would provide the kind of necessary, practical, and useful information that can help anyone intelligently decide if microdosing might be of value to them or those they love.

As you will see—and perhaps experience for yourself—*microdosing may turn out to be the most remarkable and widely used healing and wellness-enhancing modality to emerge from the current psychedelic revival.* On top of that, microdosing might give us the space, collectively, to use higher doses for spiritual and personal development, as psychedelics have been used throughout history.

Brought to You by the Worldwide Microdosing Community

This book represents the combined efforts of a worldwide community. By contributing their own experiences, thousands of individuals understood they would be helping others to make better, safer, and healthier decisions.

There are two "authors," James Fadiman and Jordan Gruber. For over a decade, I (Jim Fadiman) have been collecting, compiling, and requesting additional information from correspondents to support the growing interest in microdosing, while also exploring citizen science initiatives and reports and advising and cooperating with researchers.

Jordan and I have already written one book together, and speak with one voice. Sophia Korb created and managed the methodology and initial microdosingpsychedelics.com website, which contained basic information on substances, doses, and protocols. In return, people were asked to fill out daily checklists and submit reports. Without Sophia, microdosing might have remained my personal fixation.

Almost every description you read here was sent to my research team, or more recently, appeared in a public forum. Most of what follows are the voices of so many, from so many countries, who communicated their observations, conclusions, discoveries, and concerns about specific conditions. They were promised that their names would not be revealed, nor would they receive the credit they deserve, as the most popular microdosing substances are still illegal in most countries.

Hillary Clinton is credited for popularizing the saying "It takes a village to raise a child." In our case, it has taken a worldwide collection of villages for this book to come to fruition. Now and then, Jordan and I write about our own individual experiences, but by mainly using the editorial "we" voice, by implication we intentionally include all the many other contributors to our efforts. This book, then, is not only our way of saying "thank you" to everyone who has contributed, it is also their gift to you.

The psychedelic revival really is a big deal, and may help move us along toward saving ourselves and the environment. Microdosing often attracts far less press and attention than high-dose research and reports, but—and you can judge this for yourself—it may become a critically important and culturally accepted pathway to healing ourselves.

Meaning of Microdosing

How are "microdose" and "microdosing" defined?

"Microdose" refers to a very small dose of something. In pharmaceutical development, for example, it is one one-hundredth of a therapeutic dose, and is used to determine the safety of larger doses.[2] And as a prefix in mathematics, "micro" means one-millionth.

As for the subject of this book—microdosing psychedelics—here are the definitions used throughout:

- **Microdose** means a very small dose of a classic psychedelic (LSD, psilocybin, mescaline) and certain additional substances (including *Banisteriopsis caapi*, *Amanita muscaria*, and others) that in higher doses strongly alter consciousness.
- **Microdosing** is the practice of intermittently taking sub-threshold doses of these substances to improve creativity, boost physical energy, promote emotional balance, and increase performance on problems-solving tasks. It is also used to treat depression, anxiety, addiction, and numerous other conditions.
- **Sub-threshold** means that if you take a *correctly sized* microdose, you will not feel disoriented or intoxicated. You will not experience the effects associated with higher doses of these same substances. You won't have any substantial changes to consciousness or the way you perceive things—no psychedelic visuals or perceptions—and you won't be anywhere near a therapeutic breakthrough or a spiritually transcendent experience. During microdosing, people pursue their normal activities: work, pleasure, family, fitness, meditation, etc. However, they often report doing these activities with greater comfort and clarity.

Later in this book you will find a list of the most commonly microdosed substances. We will describe the most popular and best-researched substances, as well as others that are becoming more available and that are becoming increasingly popular.

We know we can't control the use of the term "microdosing" and that for many people, it will come to mean ingesting *any* lower-than-usual or small amount of *any* mind-altering substance on *any* schedule or even just once. But that's not what we mean, and that's not what's meant by the many people whose contributions are reflected in this book.

If you experience substantial changes in consciousness or any intoxication, you are not microdosing; if you are using substances that don't cumulatively work to produce a long-term effect in mental or physical health conditions or enhanced wellness, abilities, and flow, you are not microdosing; if you do it every day, you are not microdosing; and if it is something you take once and once only, you're not microdosing either.

Safety

Is microdosing safe? What long-term evidence is there?

This is the first question some people ask, even before learning what microdosing is, what it's for, and how to use it. And it's a good first question to ask. Physiologically, psychedelics are remarkably safe. Even massive overdoses do not result in fatalities or long-lasting major negative aftereffects. Microdoses of psychedelics—which by definition are one tenth to one twentieth or less of full doses of psychedelics—are even safer. There are, however, *a few rare conditions or situations where microdosing is contraindicated*; they are covered later in this book.

Another very common question—"Will the substance I'm microdosing interact in some way with the medication or medications I'm now using?"—is discussed in detail. An appendix of several hundred substances that are safe to use while microdosing begins on page 299.

When we ask people what they mean by "safe," a variety of specific concerns turn up. Let's look at some.

Can microdosing lower or negatively affect my quality of life? In other words, even if there might be benefits, might there also be long- or short-term physical or mental problems brought on by microdosing, as is true for many medications?

At this point, long-term reports have shown no evidence of negative effects, even if microdoses are taken over a long period of time. While there are speculations about possible long-term harm, there is no evidence to date.

Does it have any harmful short-term effects? People do report transient negative effects such as headaches, stomach discomfort, or sleep issues (usually not being able to fall asleep, but sometimes needing more sleep or needing to sleep sooner). In general, almost all the discomforts can be alleviated by lowering the size of the microdose. When this is not successful, people simply stop microdosing. No treatment or approach to health and wellness is good for everyone.

Is microdosing addictive? A substance is addictive when you need more and more of it to get the same effect, and if you stop taking it, it has physically negative symptoms. Psychedelics in general and microdosing specifically are anti-addictive in that if you take a dose too often, you develop partial or full tolerance. Eventually, you will no longer feel the effects, and taking more will make no difference. Individuals who microdose typically do so for a fixed period of time and then take time off with no negative effects.

What if I take a macrodose by mistake? If you are using reputable sources and have a good understanding of what is involved with intentionally microdosing, as described in this book, you will likely never find yourself in this situation. If you do start experiencing distinct psychedelic effects, the first thing to remember is that even very large doses of psychedelics are physically safe. Second, depending upon the situation, you may want to "go to ground"—just stay where you are or find a safe place (your home, if you can get there)—to wait out any unexpected effects. You can also reach out to someone who is experienced with psychedelics, or call a national hotline like the Fireside Project's psychedelic peer support line at **62-Fireside** (1-623-473-7433) from 11:00 AM to 11:00 PM in the US (6:00 PM to 6:00 AM GMT).

Overall, taking microdoses is far safer than taking most pharmaceuticals. Microdosing rarely negatively affects quality of life; there are generally no persistent harmful effects, and it cannot be considered addictive. Moreover, since the person who is microdosing is always in full control, they can simply discontinue microdosing if they experience any unwanted or negative effects.

Warning: Ways in Which the Word "Microdose" Is Being Misused

When Jim was determining dose sizes as part of developing the first microdosing protocol, he came up with the word "microdose," by which he meant a very small amount of LSD (measured in micrograms). The word had been invented earlier with different meanings (as discussed in chapter 6), but he didn't know that.

In the psychedelic community, the meaning of the word soon expanded to include small doses of psilocybin as well. However, by the time this manuscript reached editorial review, the word had begun to be used in all kinds of ways beyond psychedelics, usually meaning "a small amount of something," but often implying (while often not true) that whatever it was contained psychedelics.

The word "microdose" now all too often appears with no connection at all to psychedelics or how they are used. A coffee-plus-stuff product describes itself as containing a microdose of coffee. "Microdose your marriage" (whatever that might be) is now being advertised; diet pills and bikinis may be next. Bottom line: when any of us now see the word "microdose" in an advertisement, we often have no real idea what it means.

Yet many underground microdose products are indeed safe and as advertised. There is even an underground test lab that certifies them. (Yes, it's a strange world.) However, as more legal and not-yet-legal microdosing products become available, **we urge caution: read labels carefully, and do not assume that what you are told is what you get.** As for buying anything from an online source, make sure it is a legitimate company with owners you can identify, appropriate certifications and licenses, a full-fledged website presence, and so on.

Diamond Shruumz–Brand Products

A tragic misuse of the word "microdose" was made by the company selling Diamond Shruumz-brand edibles. Twenty-two kinds of products were involved, from chocolate bars to candy, many prominently displaying the word "microdose," all of which contained substances that put dozens of people in the hospital. The US FDA put out a general consumer warning as of June 20, 2024, and a full recall as of June 28, 2024. As of July 23, 2024, according to the FDA, "74 illnesses have been reported from 28 states… 38 [people] have been hospitalized, and there are two potentially associated deaths under investigation."[3]

We can hope that we won't continue to see such warnings, but the best operating principle for the foreseeable future is:

Be Careful

Do Your Research

Test Before You Taste

Why Microdose

Why do people try microdosing?

People microdose because they want to feel better, improve their health, or be better at what they do or enjoy. And many have heard or read that while there's a good chance it will make a positive difference in their lives, the cost and risk profiles remain low. The next section spells out distinct benefits that people have experienced, from improving health conditions to reducing addictions to enhancing abilities and wellness. You will also find a good deal in this book about how microdosing helps people taper and stay off pharmaceutical drugs and their undesired effects.

In a world with too much pain and dysfunction and too few resources, microdosing offers a proven tool to diminish and alleviate suffering from many physical and mental conditions. And it is generally far less expensive and much safer than pharmaceutical drugs or high-dose psychedelics.

Laboratory and animal studies show increased neuroplasticity and reduced inflammation, as well as improved functioning. People often report feeling more grounded and seeing situations and relationships more clearly, while also having more flow state experiences. At the same time, diet choices often improve, emotional resets come more easily, energy and attention levels stay focused longer, and the body often feels more relaxed and at peace.

This book is built around a compilation of personal microdosing reports—real-world evidence—in detail and with examples. We also report on media overstatements, microdosing's limitations, and other concerns, both real and theoretical.

Is it for everyone? Of course not, but most people who try it have found microdosing beneficial enough to recommend it to others. That's the main reason its use continues to spread.

Physical, Mental, and Spiritual Effects

What are the physical, mental, and spiritual benefits of microdosing?

This book includes many specific reports of medical improvements to physical and mental health. In addition, we include reports on enhanced wellness and positive effects on a wide range of other abilities (mathematics, sports, libido, food choices, and so on).

As to the benefits of microdosing, one summary comes from the Microdosing Institute of the Netherlands:[4]

Physical Benefits
Improved Sleep
More Energy
Enhanced Sensory Perception
Reduced PMS Symptoms
Decreased Pain Levels

Spiritual Benefits
Increased Sense of Wonder
Increased Sense of Unity
Deeper Emotional Connections
Greater Emotional Awareness
Increased Open-Mindedness

Mental Benefits
Improved Concentration
Increased Productivity
More Balanced Mood
More Positive Mindset

As microdosing makes good things better and bad things less bad, we divide things up more simply, into two main categories. The first is "Enhanced Abilities, Wellness, and Flow," which is where all the make-good-things-better descriptions go, and the second is "Health Conditions Positively Affected."

The kinds of claims people report—better sleep and energy; less pain and anxiety; better concentration and productivity; enhanced mood and creativity; better emotional awareness, open-mindedness, and emotional connections—are remarkable! Not everyone—or anyone in particular—will experience all, or perhaps any, of these results. However, there are some consistent patterns, so if you choose to microdose, not only might you experience some of these benefits but many people experience improvements, both with their initial concern and in areas where they were not looking for or expecting anything.

We don't yet know why microdosing catalyzes such a wide range of outcomes. Pragmatically, while we're just starting to understand the mechanisms of microdosing, we have learned a good deal about which conditions may improve with its use and how best to support any improvements.

Popularity

Why has there been such a surge in microdosing's popularity?

Let's first look at some factors that are *not* reasons (at least not yet):

- No important TikTok influencers are urging their fans to microdose.
- No large psychedelics companies are actively promoting microdosing.
- Very little research is being done by for-profit companies on microdosing.
- No major sports stars, film stars, or billionaires are promoting microdosing.
- As many media articles question the value of microdosing as talk about the benefits.
- More well-researched articles published in peer-reviewed journals are appearing, but not many, and they have not attracted much mainstream media attention.

What, then, is behind the rise of microdosing's popularity? Most likely, it is word-of-mouth recommendations from one friend to another.

The pandemic caused an increase in mental health issues worldwide. This impacted all mental health organizations and therapists, and practices were unable to expand to meet demand. At the same time, psychedelics in general—and microdosing in particular—had been reported to be helpful in dealing with loneliness, anxiety, and depression. This media buzz about microdosing—a low-cost yet effective mental health intervention—resulted in:

- An increase in microdosing organizations and individuals offering support and coaching.
- An increase in the training of new microdosing coaches internationally.
- Reports from individuals about improvements in specific conditions, especially in online forums like Reddit (which has about 275,000 people on its r/microdosing subreddit).
- Increased availability from legal sources, increased home growing, and the availability of improved psilocybin-containing mushroom "grow kits."
- Increased decriminalization throughout cities and states in the United States as well as in other countries.

In the early years of modern microdosing, from 2010 to around 2015, there had been many media stories of microdosing improving creativity, productivity, and possibly even intelligence. All these factors contributed to microdosing's initial popularity. You'll find the details of the "Beginning of Modern Microdosing" on page 272.

Concerns and Controversies

What concerns and controversies are there?

Quite a few concerns have been raised as to the short- and long-term safety of microdosing. Short-term safety concerns include the risk of an accidental overdose—taking something other than (or in addition to) what you thought you were taking—resulting in an unexpected and potentially challenging moderate or strong psychedelic experience. Another short-term risk involves potential interactions with any other medications you're taking.* Still another short-term concern is whether someone with a predisposition to certain types of mental problems could be triggered into having a full-on psychotic break, a bipolar or anxiety episode, a panic attack, and so on. We will lay out who needs to be especially careful later on.

As for long-term safety questions, critics rightly point out that we don't know for certain that microdosing is good for us—or at least that it isn't bad for us—in the long run. However, while we can't know now what we'll know 30 years from now, there have in fact been a number of studies and none of them have pointed to any long-term safety or harm concerns. For more information, see "Long-Term Safety and Impact" on page 70 and "Potential Heart Damage Concerns" on page 260.

Concerns have also been raised as to the illegality of microdosing substances in most places. At some point this will likely change, but if you are microdosing, then in many parts of the world you are doing something illegal, which necessarily exposes you to some risk. (For example, later in the book, we consider the legal anxiety and fear felt by some mothers who microdose.) Also, without full legalization and regulation, concerns about purity, standardization, and dose sizes are likely to persist.

As for dangers, from a pragmatic perspective, there are quite few. Why? Since microdosing involves taking such a tiny dose—just one tenth to one twentieth of a standard psychedelic dose, on a schedule involving regular breaks—it is remarkably safe when done correctly.

However, from the perspective of orthodox science, the safety and value of microdosing are not yet settled. We don't have that many randomized double-blind placebo-controlled studies that science likes, although there are more now than when we first started this book. We

---

*This book provides an appendix (page 299) of which substances are okay or not okay to be using if you're on a microdosing protocol.

don't ultimately know very much about the mechanisms behind how microdosing brings us to equilibrium, how it calls out our natural healing capacities, how it spurs neuroplasticity and seems to have anti-inflammatory properties, positively impacts the gut-biome axis, and so on. And while we don't fully understand the placebo effect,* we agree with the medical community that it can improve outcomes and serve as an invaluable aid to healing.

How Much Is a Microdose?

Exactly how much—how little—is a microdose?

The exact amount of a microdose varies based on the substance and whether there is a specific physical or medical condition being treated or some other wellness or performance goal. It also varies based on the bio-individuality of the person taking the substance, and how it *actually* affects them. Having said that, a microdose is usually one tenth to one twentieth of a full psychedelic dose of a substance, and leaves you in a non-intoxicated state without any psychedelic visuals or experiences.

"Sub-Perceptual"

My friends and I don't think microdosing is sub-perceptual. What gives?

You are correct that describing microdosing effects as "sub-perceptual" is, at best, incomplete and misleading. (The term "sub-perceptible" is now often used.) Here is an explanation, an alternative, and an apology.

In first attempting to describe microdosing, the goal was to find a word that indicated that it did not have any of the effects of a classic psychedelic.

---

*The placebo *effect* can also be thought of in terms of the innate ability of the mind to facilitate the release and use of natural healing factors and abilities that are built into all human beings. It is part of how human beings are constituted, an *innate process or capacity* that—through certain types of thinking, feeling, and nervous system regulation—accelerates healing. We agree that there are placebo and expectations effects involved with microdosing, but we also now have scientific proof that it is not *only* placebo and expectations.

"Sub-psychedelic effects" sounded terrible, and "sub-hallucinogenic" wasn't an option because psychedelics don't cause actual hallucinations as they are technically defined.* "Sub-perceptual" was not a great choice, but it at least alerted people to stop looking for visual changes, visions, visits from divine spirits, flowers on wallpaper smiling at you, and the like.

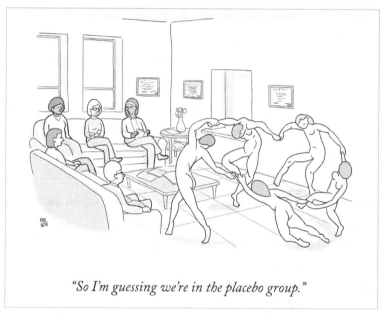

"So I'm guessing we're in the placebo group."

By @paulnoth in @altajournal (2023)

A better term may be "sub-threshold," that is, below the threshold of a psychedelic experience. People experienced in taking high doses understand the term "sub-threshold," and it sounds like it means something to those who haven't had such experiences. It doesn't say exactly *what* it's a threshold of—just that the effects are below that. For our purposes, however, it means below the threshold of a psychedelic

---

*Hallucinations seem real, but they are not. *"Hallucinations are where you hear, see, smell, taste or feel things that appear to be real but only exist in your mind"* (National Health Service, United Kingdom). Eyes open or closed, people who report visual and sensory changes while using high doses of psychedelics may appreciate or be disturbed by their visions, but do not think of them as *actual* landscapes, physical objects, or sounds. While one of the older inaccurate terms for psychedelics is "hallucinogens," attributing this kind of reality misapprehension to them is simply inaccurate.

experience, both perceptually and experientially. There are no major changes in how reality is perceived and no intoxication. You may have more energy, colors may appear a little brighter and sounds a little clearer, and you may notice you are thinking more creatively or better able to focus. But that's about as far as it goes.

The apology is from Jim:

As the first to have used the term, I've been unable to stop its spread, or its morphing into "sub-perceptible." Given that mistakes and misinformation last on the internet forever, "sub-perceptual" will continue to appear long after I'm gone. Please accept my apologies. Good for you for having the good sense to question what you have read when it doesn't match your experience.

The best concise description of this dynamic comes from an excellent review of microdosing research by Genís Ona and José Carlos Bouso (2020): "Thus, although subtle, the effects of microdosing psychedelics are noticeable."[5]

Reasons for Some People Not to Microdose

Let's look at a few categories:

Preexisting Physical Conditions: None have been noted, except tinnitus and red-green color blindness.

In healthy individuals, one concern is that *tinnitus* (a continual ringing, noise, or other sound in the ears) sometimes becomes worse while microdosing. In almost every case, the level of tinnitus has gone back to what it had been before, or even less, when the microdosing was stopped. Some individuals have also reported tinnitus for the first time while microdosing, but it went away soon after they stopped.

When looking away from a light source, people with red-green color blindness report tracers—blurs or streaks of light trailing behind moving objects—for up to several days after microdosing. We've suggested for some years that they not microdose. In response, we've since received reports such as, "Yes, I had tracers, but the overall benefits were worth it." Make your own decision. Most minor physical complaints—including these visual problems as well as sleep disturbances—were alleviated when people reduced their dose size.

Mental Health: Should you find microdosing too uncomfortable or disturbing in any way, first cut the dose size in half, and if that doesn't help, simply stop entirely.

Motivation: As with any other activity that you engage in, placing close attention on what you intend or desire will probably improve the outcome. Many people also discover improvements in conditions they were not focused on.

Expectations and Placebo: Conventional wisdom correctly holds that positive expectations improve our body's natural healing response. This principle is so well established that every available method for increasing the anticipation of positive and beneficial results—such as setting positive expectations, emphasizing the likelihood of success, and cultivating a warm trusting consultative manner—should be deployed by conventional medical practitioners, by psychotherapists, and certainly by high-dose psychedelic session leaders.

Legal Concerns: While legal restrictions against using psychedelics are generally diminishing throughout the world, they still exist. Anyone who uses any of these substances in any amount for self-development or healing should be aware of the real-time legal status of the substance. One resource to start with is the "Psychedelic Legalization & Decriminalization Tracker" at psychedelicalpha.com/data/psychedelic-laws for the United States and the "Worldwide Psychedelic Laws Tracker" at psychedelicalpha.com/data/worldwide-psychedelic-laws for the rest of the world.

Quality and Purity: The most frequent answer to the question of how to verify the quality and purity of any particular substance is to obtain a testing kit. More recently, there has been a rise in recommendations to grow one's own psilocybin mushrooms. In addition, there are a growing number of companies selling a variety of substances online (often illegally). We will return to these questions later.

Value of Hesitation

When something gets this popular this fast, I see yellow flags and warning lights. Should I still proceed?

It's a wonderful question and impossible to answer, a bit like asking the question, "Can you please give me a list of all the people who were not invited to the party?"

For some people, the extent to which microdosing has become so widely known and used automatically suggests it may be a fad, unrealistically hyped, or perhaps even fraudulent. For example, a prominent researcher (discussed in chapter 6) has noted that the closer we get to ideal scientific experimental conditions, the less it seems possible to demonstrate any effect from microdosing. But still, we are struck that so many individuals who freely chose how and when to microdose, and who gained nothing by doing so, have favorably reported about their microdosing experiences.

This book includes very few reports from people who did not have a good experience, or who quit soon after they began. Maybe they did so because they were uncomfortable and assumed that their only option was to stop rather than to seek advice to see if they were microdosing correctly. There are many possible reasons, including someone doing everything exactly right and simply not feeling any benefits. (In most research studies, those who drop out are the ones you *most* want to speak to, as they can best tell you about the limitations of your work.)

So, dear questioner, if your concerns are strong enough to prevent you from microdosing, that in itself is a good and sufficient reason not to do so. There's a Chinese saying, "The journey of a thousand miles begins with a single step." If, for any reason—real or imagined, justified or ridiculous, studiously arrived at or frivolously decided—you don't take that single step, then the journey for you is just over. That's fine, and you can simply move on.

Over many decades, Jim has been buttonholed by people who say, "I'm thinking of taking LSD, but . . ." Jim interrupts them: "I wouldn't do it, then." They often persist in wanting to tell him why they are hesitating. His position remains that hesitating for any reason is reason enough not to take the first step. The quality of the reason is irrelevant and of course we're free to change our minds in the future.

What's impressive about so many of the people you will meet in this book is their actual reporting on how microdosing worked for them: a lot, somewhat, a little, barely, or not at all. They shared their experiences so that other people could learn from them.

We are strongly supportive of people not microdosing without needing to give any justification. For those of you who share the concerns of this questioner, it's better for you to wait—perhaps to get more information, advice, or life experience—but *definitely do not proceed* if your sense of inner caution tells you not to.

Legality

Where is—and isn't—microdosing legal?

Legality is and for now will continue to be a moving target, depending on the legal status of the underlying substance being used. In most countries, and in most US states and cities, microdosing is still illegal with regard to most substances. What's most important is that you have an accurate understanding of the legal rules—*as they are actually enforced*—within the jurisdiction and the legal climate where you live.

Finding Substances

Can this book help me find substances for microdosing?

No. It is a curious world we live in where the act of making a desired substance illegal almost overnight creates a worldwide illegal market for said substance. Therefore, if you live in a part of the world where the substances are not yet legal, you're on your own.

What we find over and over again, however, is that in a world of increasingly available information and connection, people eventually find a way. Many of the substances discussed in this book are plants or fungi that can be found growing naturally, or which can be easily cultivated. Asking friends and joining psychedelic interest groups and taking classes or growing your own psilocybin-containing mushrooms are all options.

In the US, the pressure is increasing on legislatures and regulatory agencies to do something. Burdened by growing numbers of citizens who could benefit from psychedelics in general—and from microdosing in particular—they are looking for ways to make psychedelics available, either through medical institutions and practitioners, or by loosening or rescinding current legal restrictions. This issue becomes increasingly irrelevant as the whole idea of preventing people from having access to safe and effective substances that lessen suffering and improve functioning becomes seen as more and more ridiculous.

What Doctors, Therapists, Coaches, and Other Professionals Need to Know

To begin with, medical professionals are sharply limited in what they are allowed to do. If they violate any laws, regulations, or special restrictions agreed upon by the local, state, or national organizations that oversee them, they can lose their license and be charged with criminal offenses. Similarly, in their training, because of these restrictions, they will generally not have been taught even basic information and ways of improving safety and efficacy when using psychedelics. This is changing, but slowly.

This book is limited to understanding and working with microdoses for individuals. There are a growing number of organizations that offer training about psychedelics, how they can be used effectively, contraindications, etc. Most of this information, geared to professionals, still focuses on high-dose use. This makes sense, as almost all the negative reports related to using psychedelics arise from difficult high-dose events.

We have many reports of therapists of many types, encouraged either by their own experiences or what they hear back from their clients about microdosing, making an effort to learn as much as they can. As the laws become more realistic, there is a growing need for professionals to have personal psychedelic experience as well as training in helping others.

"Coaching" is a term we use in this book. It suggests less intrusion—and more support and listening—from a therapist or other medical professional. In the psychotherapeutic community it is becoming recognized that clients who microdose—with or without their therapist's support—"do better." That means that they make progress faster and are much more able to directly look at upsetting issues. They are better able to make use of therapeutic suggestions and interventions. This book does not take the place of real-world training from qualified and experienced supervisors or mentors.

Making Best Use of This Book

At public presentations on different applications of microdosing, we've often heard: "I had no idea that you could microdose for *that*."

With very few exceptions, new waves of psychedelic research—and the stated uses for different psychedelics described by literally hundreds of companies attempting to sell a molecule, a treatment, a franchise, or a mix of those—have focused on mental conditions.

This book explores many more possibilities as reported by individuals from around the world who have been helped by microdosing, including improvements with physically based conditions like shingles, multiple sclerosis, pain, and much more. Reading over the wide range of actual reported results will encourage you to remember that, while mental and physical health may represent different occupational specializations, you are a unified mental/physical being, which means that improvements in one area are very often matched by improvements in others.

Moreover, while most of the scientific and clinical research (and funding) on psychedelics generally and microdosing in particular focuses on illness, we will be covering the larger realm of improved well-being—of exceeding previous real or imagined limitations—as well as enhanced abilities in a wide variety of realms.

We don't—and can't—know what's possible for you, but what we do know is that there are many useful tools, foods, practices, supplements, and mental states that, for some people, are truly beneficial. Perhaps the best way to get the most from this book is to consider it like an all-purpose handle that can be inserted into many different tools. Along with duct tape, WD-40, good sleep, healthy eating, exercise, and good relationships, the information in this book can become part of your daily "Get-More-Out-Of-This-Life" kit.

[2]

Basics

This chapter provides information you'll want to have at your disposal should you decide to begin (or further) your exploration of microdosing. The following areas will be covered:

- **Substances:** What substances are people using, how do they differ, and are they legal?
- **How Taken/What With:** How and with what do people actually consume microdoses?
- **Dosage Range:** What's the right dose range for each substance? When does this change?
- **Protocols:** What schedule should you microdose with, and when should you take breaks?
- **Safety and Other Concerns:** What the concerns are; staying safe and sound.
- **Best Practices/Outside Guidance:** What often works well for people; when to seek outside help.
- **Health Conditions Preliminaries:** Information applying to all health conditions covered herein.

Substances Used for Microdosing

The great majority of people who microdose take either LSD or psilocybin-containing mushrooms. These classic psychedelics are the most researched, the best described, and—although not yet legal in most countries—the most readily available. They are physically safe at high doses, and even safer taken as microdoses. The following list includes other substances that are being used for microdosing, including those that are sometimes spoken of in microdosing terms and those that are simply not recommended.

Widely Microdosed
- psilocybin
- LSD

Also Microdosed
- Illegal in the US, legal in many other countries
  » peyote, ayahuasca, ALD-52, 1p-LSD
- Legal in the US and most other countries
  » *Amanita muscaria* (a mushroom)
  » *Banisteriopsis caapi* (the vine component of ayahuasca)
  » LSA—morning glory seeds, Hawaiian baby woodrose seeds
  » San Pedro and other cactuses*

Sometimes Spoken Of in Microdosing Terms
- cannabis
- DMT
- ibogaine

---

*Alexandra Hicks tells us there are roughly three hundred cactus species that contain mescaline and other mind-altering alkaloids. Most have not been studied (Hicks, 2023).

Not Recommended for Microdosing

- MDMA
- *Salvia divinorum*
- ketamine

In this book, we focus on the extensive microdosing reports we've received on psilocybin and LSD. Over time, as increasing numbers of people microdose with other substances, we'll be able to update the above list. For example, since the publication of the first extensive study on *Amanita muscaria* (Masha, 2022), reports are starting to come in about its uses. When appropriate, we refer to *Amanita muscaria*'s benefits for certain conditions.

As for MDMA, *Salvia divinorum,* ibogaine, and ketamine, while we are aware of enthusiastic individuals and groups using small doses of these substances and calling what they're doing "microdosing," we do not recommend them for microdosing based on how they're used—including the difficulties of assessing a proper dose size—and the types of results reported. They simply run too far afield from the main focus of this book, or we have too little information.

Let's briefly review two substances characterized as "sometimes spoken of in microdosing terms"—DMT and cannabis.

DMT: Vape pens (and intranasal sprays) for "microdosing DMT" are increasingly available and popular. These vape pens (whether N,N-DMT or 5-MeO-DMT) are designed to titrate the intensity of one of the strongest psychedelics known. While touted for immediately reducing anxiety, the intense short-duration effects of DMT—even when "microdosed" in this relatively controlled fashion—easily lead to intoxication or euphoria. Plus, a desire to have more immediately after the initial effect wears off is not uncommon. So, while people may be speaking of "microdosing DMT," they are actually describing taking very small individual doses, with no protocols, time between, or time off. Not microdosing, just brief pleasant conscious-altering experiences.

Cannabis: To speak about "microdosing" cannabis (marijuana) is a misuse of the term. The mechanisms, biology, and effects of cannabis are unique, complex, and powerful, but it does not resemble microdosing substances nor does its use provide the same range of benefits.

Microdosing specifically refers to taking very small amounts of a psychedelic on a specific schedule over a number of weeks. The same term applied to taking a little bit of cannabis has nothing to do with actual microdosing. The effects and benefits of cannabis are totally different from the effects of psychedelics. Cannabis—the whole plant and a number of its different alkaloids—has been used successfully as a medication for many conditions. Good books on "medical marijuana" are available.[1]

Cannabis acts on and through the endocannabinoid system and affects the brain, body, and whole being differently than substances like LSD and psilocybin. Cannabis generally impedes neuroplasticity rather than enhances it. Brumback et al. (2016) conclude that "THC appears to block synaptic plasticity and neurogenesis"—the exact opposite of microdosing's effects. Conor Murray's 2024 research, discussed on page 236, showed that LSD increased neural complexity, but THC did not.

Cannabis is generally not taken with any standard protocol (days on/days off). People report "microdosing" cannabis throughout the day. None of this is microdosing.

Moreover, THC is fat soluble and stores in the body's fatty tissues and is detectable weeks after one stops using it. LSD and psilocybin are gone from the body within a day or so. Effective protocols are not possible because of this persistence. Conscious use of very small amounts of cannabis can be a rewarding experience or valuable practice, but it's not microdosing.

Other Substances

Are substances beyond the "classic" psychedelics being used?

When modern microdosing started taking off in the early 2010s, the focus was nearly exclusively on LSD and psilocybin-containing mushrooms, two of the "classic psychedelics" (the other two are mescaline and DMT). Based on work with these substances, the Fadiman protocol (or schedule) and other protocols were developed, reports were received from thousands of people, and the general outlines of modern microdosing came into being.

Today, the range of substances being used (and the way in which they are being used) has expanded. When this book was initially conceived in 2020, little information was available on microdosing *Amanita muscaria*. Since then, Baba Masha's book *Microdosing with Amanita Muscaria* (2022) came out, and we started to hear stories of people benefiting from this mushroom when *properly prepared and used*. That's why this book includes it as a (generally legal) microdosing substance, even though it is not considered a classic psychedelic because it works primarily with the GABA and not the serotonin system.

On the other hand, when a substance—even at the lowest of doses—is potentially dangerous, addictive, or disorienting, or usually brings about some level of immediate intoxication or disorientation, it's not for microdosing. For example, smoking *Salvia divinorum* often produces immediate disorientation, no matter how small the dose.

LSD

What's important to know?

> I did not choose LSD; LSD found and called me.
> —Albert Hofmann

Lysergic acid diethylamide, LSD-25, is the best-known psychedelic and the one most associated with 1960s counterculture. First synthesized in 1938 by Albert Hofmann, it was the twenty-fifth lysergic acid derivative he'd created. He noted that it "produced some restlessness in mice"—but little else—and it was put aside.

However, in 1943 Hofmann had an intuition that LSD-25 might

have other possibilities. He resynthesized it and, in so doing, inadvertently absorbed some, perhaps through a cut on his finger. Puzzled and disturbed by how he felt soon after, he went home and observed some hours of unusual feelings and images. The next day, guessing the LSD-25 had been the cause, he took what he felt would be the smallest possible dose that would have any noticeable effect—250 micrograms—actually a substantial dose.

His own description of his remarkable experience, including both ecstatic and frightening periods, has been widely published. LSD attracted initial interest because, even at doses of just fifty or one hundred millionths of a gram, it induced extreme altered states. Sandoz Pharmaceuticals, Hofmann's employer, hoped there would be some commercial use for a substance with such powerful effects at such a tiny dose. They distributed it freely and urged researchers to experiment with it and report their findings. The effects of microdoses were overlooked, in part because the smallest dose that Sandoz shipped was twenty-five micrograms. According to Jim:

> By the time I was introduced to LSD in 1961, it was the most widely researched psychiatric drug in the world. I wrote Sandoz and asked for any published research on LSD. I received two huge volumes from Switzerland which contained abstracts of the first thousand published papers. In 1970, solely for political reasons (not for scientific or medical reasons), the US government declared, without evidence, that along with other psychedelics, LSD had no medical uses and a potential for abuse. Regulations then made these substances almost impossible to research and illegal to manufacture, distribute, or possess.

LSD is still illegal in most places. In the US, even with the current resurgence of interest—with many research centers using it, and with increasing amounts of public and scientific attention being paid to it—the Food and Drug Administration has not yet changed its classification.

Not surprisingly, once it was restricted worldwide, a black market for LSD sprang into existence and has remained active ever since. LSD is usually sold either as individual doses on a sheet of blotter paper—scored into tiny squares, often imprinted with a design—or in liquid form in very small bottles. In the past few years, lower doses, especially for microdosing, have become available in both forms.

Surprising fact: One microgram of pure LSD (one millionth of a gram) contains 1.54 quadrillion (1,540,000,000,000,000) molecules.[2] The most common LSD microdose size—ten micrograms, or just over 15 quadrillion molecules—is enough to potentially affect all relevant brain and body cells many times over. (LSD likely affects around 10% of the body's cells; human males have around 36 trillion cells, females 28 trillion, and children 17 trillion.[3])

Current status: In the US, LSD is still legally unavailable, except for research, even in states or cities that have decriminalized naturally occurring psychedelics. Most companies working with psychedelics have focused their attention on other molecules.

Psilocybin "Magic" Mushrooms

What are the important facts to know?

Psilocybin is found in almost two hundred species of *Psilocybe* mushrooms, which grow on every continent except Antarctica. Many species thrive in animal dung as well as in disturbed soil moved around by agriculture or construction. Popular species are now cultivated by individuals, indoors and out. In Holland, while the fruiting body (the mushroom) is not legal, truffles (technically, the "sclerotia")—which grow underground just before the mushroom breaks through the surface—are legal. The mycelium, a network of ultrafine root threads, also contains psilocybin as well as other alkaloids, and some companies now directly harvest the mycelium.

Currently in the US, while psilocybin-containing mushrooms, truffles, and mycelium are all restricted under federal and most state laws, it is legal in forty-eight of the fifty states to order a spore print of any psilocybin species. A spore print is a method of taking and storing spores from mushrooms. Spores can be thought of as fungal seeds. Mushrooms reproduce by spores, and a spore print is simply what one gets by putting a mushroom onto a sterile surface, such as aluminum foil, and letting it sit overnight, allowing the spores to fall onto the surface.

There is also laboratory-grown psilocybin—from a yeast—and other relatively inexpensive methods of synthesis are now available in the public domain. Proprietary methods of synthesizing psilocybin exist, but these are rarely used by those interested in microdosing. Most clinical and laboratory published research on psilocybin has been done with laboratory-generated psilocybin. Almost all microdosing reported in this book has been done with dried whole mushrooms, which aren't completely comparable.

To date, there are only a few animal studies comparing isolated psilocybin and natural psilocybin in the whole mushroom. In those studies, whole psilocybin including its entourage compounds was significantly more effective.[4]

Legal status: "The legal status of unauthorized [use of] psilocybin mushrooms varies worldwide."[5] Enforcement varies widely as well. A few countries, like Jamaica, Brazil, and Nepal, have no restrictions. Others, like Italy and Portugal, have decriminalized psilocybin, and many countries, like India, Vietnam, and Thailand, have legal restrictions that generally go unenforced.

As decriminalization spreads to more US states and cities, and as more robust legalization occurs, psilocybin-containing mushrooms, measured and packaged for purity and stability, will become increasingly available. Homegrown cultivation continues to proliferate.

Surprising fact: Psilocybin itself is not very psychoactive, if at all. Once consumed, it is converted, primarily by the liver, into psilocin. Psilocin, in turn, is the molecule responsible for most psychoactive properties of magic mushrooms. Psilocybin is stable, psilocin less so.

Not as surprising a fact: Other alkaloids found in psychedelic mushrooms include norpsilocin, baeocystin, norbaeocystin, and aerugina-scin. We know very little about their individual effects.

Illegal/Legal

Why are magic mushrooms and LSD generally illegal, but San Pedro cactuses and Amanita muscaria legal?

We'll break that question into three parts:

- Why are magic mushrooms and LSD illegal?
- Why is San Pedro cactus legal?
- Why is the mushroom *Amanita muscaria* legal?

In a sensible world, with legislation based on accurate information and the public's needs, psilocybin-containing mushrooms, LSD, and a host of other consciousness-altering substances would not be illegal, and in the future perhaps they won't be. The original legislation that banned these substances was pushed through Congress without any input from appropriate scientific and regulatory agencies, and was intended to give President Nixon a way to attack individuals and organizations whom he personally disliked or who publicly spoke out against some of his policies.* So they were placed on Schedule I, and according to the Drug Enforcement Administration's (DEA's) current website[6]:

> Schedule I drugs, substances, or chemicals are defined as drugs
> with no currently accepted medical use and a high potential for

---

*According to John Ehrlichman, Assistant to the President for Domestic Affairs under President Richard Nixon: "'You want to know what this was really all about?' he [Ehrlichman] asked with the bluntness of a man who, after public disgrace and a stretch in federal prison, had little left to protect. 'The Nixon campaign in 1968, and the Nixon White House after that, had two enemies: the antiwar left and black people. You understand what I'm saying? We knew we couldn't make it illegal to be either against the war or black, but by getting the public to associate the hippies with marijuana [and LSD] and blacks with heroin, and then criminalizing both heavily, we could disrupt those communities. We could arrest their leaders, raid their homes, break up their meetings, and vilify them night after night on the evening news. *Did we know we were lying about the drugs? Of course we did*'" (Turner, 2018).

abuse. Some examples of Schedule I drugs are: heroin, lysergic acid diethylamide (LSD), marijuana (cannabis), 3,4-methylene-dioxymethamphetamine (ecstasy), methaqualone, and peyote.

This disconnect from reality was as clear at the time of its passage in 1970 as it is now. At the time LSD was scheduled, it was the most researched psychiatric drug in the world, and at least forty thousand people had been given it safely in research and clinical settings with much the same results that current research shows. Cannabis was included to give Nixon the tool to attack some of the other groups he disliked. MDMA (or "Ecstasy," as the government calls it) was added later when it became a popular recreational drug. It had already been used by a large number of therapists, especially those working with couples. Originally known as "Adam" for its ability to bring about a perceived innocence and natural state, it proved particularly useful in facilitating emotional openness and communication, and was typically offered by licensed therapists who found it so effective they were willing to take the chance of losing their license or going to jail if found out.

Peyote, a small slow-growing cactus, was little known outside the Native American community. It was probably added because it contains the alkaloid mescaline, which has similar effects to LSD. San Pedro cactus, which also contains mescaline and has been used ritually and for healing purposes by indigenous peoples in parts of South America for centuries, was not put on Schedule I. This is probably because whoever wrote up the original bill didn't know about it, and since it was not widely used in the United States, nobody thought to add it.

The simple answer, then, is that there is no good reason for any psychedelic substances to have been put onto Schedule I in the first place. Now, there is far less reason to keep them there given the great number of positive medical research findings associated with psychedelics of all kinds, not to mention the explosion of potential commercial opportunities and uses for mental health and other issues.

A few years ago, an inquiry into the availability of psychedelic plants or fungi on Amazon.com produced some interesting results. San Pedro cactus was available on dozens of sites as were Hawaiian baby woodrose seeds and morning glory seeds, with commercial names like "Pearly Gates" and "Heavenly Blue." These contain LSA (lysergic acid amide), which has identical properties to LSD but at roughly a hundredth the strength.

In short, the restrictions on the use of psilocybin, LSD, peyote, and later MDMA were political, not medical or psychological. San Pedro cactus escaped being scheduled simply by not being noticed. *Amanita muscaria* was never considered to be on any schedule, and is just now being recognized for microdosing. In most mushroom identification books, *Amanita muscaria* will be listed as toxic, and indeed it can be if consumed raw or taken in large quantities.

LSD and Psilocybin Differences

What's the difference between psilocybin and LSD?

This is among the most frequently asked questions. Early on in his research, Jim's colleague Sophia Korb reviewed reports from the "vaults" of the Erowid.org website—one hundred experiences with LSD, and one hundred with psilocybin. They were all high-dose experiences, which were presumed to be more likely than microdoses to show differences. Appropriate software, programmed to ignore the words "LSD" and "psilocybin" during its analysis, searched the descriptions. It was *not* able to distinguish LSD-generated reports from psilocybin-generated ones, beyond the well-known and obvious time differences in major effects.*

Several studies have looked at the differences between LSD and synthesized psilocybin but did not find any in their effects on physiology or cognition, except that the effects lasted longer with LSD. For

---

*LSD effects typically last 8–12 hours, those of psilocybin 4–6 hours.

microdosing purposes, the science shows it is realistic to treat the two substances as mainly identical when dose levels are matched.

However, we now also have thousands of written reports and survey reports based on actual microdosing. These real-world reports agree as to differences between the two substances.

A young man in Los Angeles summed it up: "My friends, who have been microdosing and high-dosing with LSD and psilocybin over the past few years, generally agree that psilocybin is a warmer and friendlier experience, while LSD is more analytic and objective—better for thinking than feeling." Another report concluded: "LSD microdoses are more energetic and provide reliable focused energy, while mushrooms are better for working with your heart and emotions."

It may be that the entourage compounds (in addition to the psilocybin) in mushrooms help to more directly bring forth emotions and even traumas, making mushrooms the preferable microdosing substance for such issues. Also, it's not uncommon with mushrooms, even at microdosing levels, for people to feel a connection to or the presence of a being or entity of some kind.

Whatever the distinctions may be between LSD and psilocybin-containing mushrooms, their effects on improving health and enhancing healthy functioning are generally similar. As the psychedelic microdosing world opens up, and more people start working with more substances—including *Amanita muscaria,* ayahuasca, San Pedro, and perhaps the iboga shrub (or ibogaine, an alkaloid derived from it)—better ways of working with each substance are being tested and developed.

How Microdoses Are Taken (and What With)

How do people usually take microdoses of LSD or psilocybin-containing mushrooms?

LSD: LSD often comes as fifty or one hundred micrograms on a tiny tab of very light cardboard, often a quarter-inch square. A whole sheet of these tabs often has a pattern or image printed on it. (See Erik Davis's book *Blotter: The Untold Story of an Acid Medium* [2024].) Dropping a tab in a measured amount of distilled water, water with vodka, or just vodka, is the most accurate and commonly used microdosing method. For example, if a tab has one hundred micrograms dissolved in one hundred drops of liquid measured from a dropper, each drop will have one microgram of LSD. This method is known as "volumetric measurement," meaning you are measuring the volume of liquid.

Far less accurate—but people really do this—is to attempt to cut the tab into equal pieces so that one tiny piece can then be put on the tongue. This is not recommended for obvious reasons.

LSD can also come in a small amount of liquid, with each drop containing ten to one hundred micrograms (or more). In this instance, one or more drops may be put into a liquid, as above, so similar measurements can be made.

Psilocybin-containing mushrooms: More and more often, these are sold in premeasured capsules, sometimes with additional substances in the capsule. (See the discussion of "stacking" in the next answer.) If the dose you want is less than what is in the capsule, open it, pour out the powder in a thin line, then divide it up for accurate measurement. Fresh mushrooms should be dried, ground into powder, and put into capsules or taken in tea or other liquid. (See lemon-tekking later in this chapter.) You will need a scale that can measure hundredths of a gram, which are available online for about $20 US.

If you are using "truffles," follow the directions from the vendor, and see our general rules of thumb in the "Dose Levels for Other Substances" section on page 46.

Combinations and Stacking

What other kinds of substances are people taking with their microdoses?

Many different kinds of things are being tried and experimented with. How each one, singly or as part of a group, affects microdosing is largely uncharted territory. We will limit our answer to a few examples and some general trends.

Indigenous people worldwide have used microdoses of consciousness-altering substances singly and as part of mixtures. For example, the Aztecs, at the time of first contact with the Spanish, were mixing cacao (what chocolate is made from) and psilocybin mushrooms for celebrations and quiet contemplations. Today, there are microdosing coaches who work with psilocybin and "ceremonial cacao." According to one source:

> The combination of sacred mushrooms and cacao share a long history and tradition. Traditionally used in ceremonies with larger dose journeys, we like to propose this combination for microdosing too. Separately cacao and microdosing are used for a healthy and positive lifestyle, together they give more depth. Cacao is not a psychedelic, but it does have a psychoactive effect as a mood enhancer.[7]

Promoted by Paul Stamets, "stacking" has gained widespread popularity and refers to combining psilocybin with substances of any kind. The "Stamets stack" combines a microdose of psilocybin, an equivalent amount of lion's mane mushroom, and a small amount of flushing niacin (vitamin B3).* Stamets proposed that this combination improves cognitive functioning, with the niacin dilating blood vessels and improving the delivery of other substances throughout the body.

As part of a recent massive study, thousands of individuals from more than eighty countries contributed to a survey of microdosing use.[8] Individuals taking the "Stamets stack" had higher scores on some measures of cognitive improvement and flexibility than individuals who microdosed without additional substances. "Tap test" scores—based

---

*Most vitamin B3 that is produced, sold, and consumed is of the non-flushing variety. If you do take flushing niacin, you will experience the equivalent of a light sunburn: your skin will tingle, it may redden or darken a little, and you may be a bit uncomfortable. The effect goes away within a half hour to two hours and causes no harm, but many find it uncomfortable.

on how quickly someone can tap a finger on a surface or two fingers together, usually for ten seconds*—showed that those who microdosed performed better than those who didn't, and those who used the "Stamets stack" outperformed the other two groups.

A microdose coach whose clients include individuals recovering from traumatic brain injury and addiction sends his clients capsules with four different mushrooms, which they add to their psilocybin to enhance its effectiveness. He reports that after microdosing for a period of time, some of his clients (whose improvements have continued) indicate they are taking *only* the functional mushrooms.

There are herbalists experimenting with mixtures of various herbs along with psilocybin. Western medicine is particularly weak in its ability to analyze complicated mixes of substances, so it's not surprising that two of the talented herbalists we know of have been trained in Chinese medicine, which has been developing herbal tonics for more than a thousand years. It's of course difficult to determine the results of such complex mixtures, but one of these herbalists reports that everyone who has used her herbal elixir preferred it to psilocybin alone.

One addition to microdosing psilocybin, called "lemon-tekking," is the addition of lemon juice at the time of ingestion. This has moved from anecdotal and historical uses to having the proven present-day effects described below.

Undoubtedly, with wider legalization and decriminalization, expanding research, and the possibility of creating profitable products all marching along and feeding off each other, we will eventually see a profusion of "microdose plus" concoctions.

---

*Finger tapping and "speed tapping" apps are available for smartphones.

Lemon-Tekking

What is "lemon-tekking," and how does it relate to microdosing?

"Lemon-tekking"* means pouring lemon juice—which has a low pH (very acidic)—over a dose of psilocybin-containing mushrooms that has already been ground into a powder.† Enough lemon juice is used to saturate the powder. After the mushrooms soak in the lemon juice for about twenty-five minutes, the combination is consumed, adding more water or just as a single shot. It can also be added to tinctures or tea. Lemon-tekking accelerates the liver's conversion of psilocybin, which the body can't directly use, into psilocin, which is biologically active.[9] There are three main results:

- The acidic lemon juice makes it easier to swallow and digest the mushroom generally, helping overcome discomfort for those who otherwise can't easily handle the taste of mushrooms or feel any discomfort in eating, swallowing, and processing them.
- The overall experience has a quicker onset and a shorter overall duration, sometimes by an hour or more.
- By speeding the conversion of psilocybin to psilocin, the experience often comes on not just more quickly but more intensely. For those with weak liver functioning or other digestive or absorption problems, lemon-tekking makes a big difference.

More popular for larger doses, lemon-tekking can also be applied to microdosing. Even at the recommended dose level for psilocybin-containing mushrooms, for those who feel any discomfort, lemon-

---

*"Tekking" is derived from "technique."

†Mushroom dust should not be inhaled, so always wear a mask before beginning any grinding.

tekking can help. If, however, lemon-tekking intensifies your experience beyond what is comfortable, it's best to lower the dose. Some people report that they always lemon-tek their microdoses, adjusting their dose accordingly, perhaps starting with only half as much.

Onset

How soon will one feel effects when microdosing?

People sometimes notice effects of a microdose within the first thirty minutes to an hour, while for others it takes up to a few hours, and still others hardly experience anything at all. Changes in behavior, thinking, healing, and feeling often occur only after being on a protocol for a period of time, but important insights or health changes can occur even on the first day. Consider these two submitted reports.

- "The first capsule I took in the morning, I was very cynical on whether or not this would actually work. But after about 30 mins I felt like a weight was slowly lifting off my shoulders. I found things just a tiny bit more beautiful (my potted plants for example had never looked so beautiful) and I suddenly felt the urge to water them all and make sure they were okay. Also, the first day things were really gorgeous, not trippy, just prettier. I even saw a sort of rainbow-colored cloud for a second, but these visual effects didn't really continue after the first capsule, it was just the first."
- "I tried my first microdose today, about six hours ago, and thought my initial experiences would help others. (I've been on and off antidepressants for 20 years.) I took about .05 grams of Psilocybe Mexicana. What I'm really aware of is that there have been no chains of obsessive unwanted thoughts or thoughts that led to a downward spiral of negative thinking."

Dosage Ranges for Different Substances

How did the recommended dose levels arise?

As is true more often than you might expect in science, the initial recommended dose was based on a mistake. In 2010, during lunch in a Greek restaurant in Santa Cruz, California, Robert Forte told Jim that Albert Hofmann had taken very low doses, which he felt were very beneficial. (True.*) According to Jim:

> My recollection is that Robert said "10 micrograms," but that's either my misremembering or mishearing, as he likely said "20 micrograms." I found this out later, talking to Hofmann's biographer and several of his close personal friends.

The reality is that twenty micrograms of LSD is typically way too much for microdosing. At this level, psychedelic effects become noticeable, and some intoxication is possible. Had twenty micrograms been the initial instruction given to Jim's early self-reporters, modern microdosing might have still happened, but it would likely have unfolded later on and differently.

What evolved from the first round of reports was that approximately a tenth to a twentieth of a recreational dose produced positive effects, but none of the signature changes in consciousness or perception asso-

---

*Hofmann had told people that he regretted that Sandoz Pharmaceuticals had never explored very low doses. He had personally experimented with very low doses of LSD much earlier in his life while doing Swiss military service. In an interview with several psychedelic researchers during his hundredth birthday celebration, he and Rick Doblin, the founder of MAPS, had the following dialogue (Hofmann et al., 2005, 91–92):

Rick: I remember a while ago, you said one of the most unexplored areas of research with LSD was low doses.

Albert: Yes, that would be interesting . . .

Rick: What kind of doses are you talking about, when you would go out walking?

Albert: Twenty-five micrograms, twenty-five instead of 125. Or even lower: ten.

Rick: Wow. Can you actually notice when you take ten micrograms? Can you notice that you've taken it?

Albert: Oh, yes! Yes. An improved response to nature. Improved experience of nature, yes. And of thinking, a big improvement in thinking.

At that point in time, there was no further follow-up on Hofmann's suggestion.

ciated with a full dose of a classic psychedelic. These days, most people find the correct dose range is either a little higher or a little lower than ten micrograms of LSD, or between one and three tenths of a gram of psilocybin, and an accordingly small dose level for other substances that are being microdosed.

This fortunate initial mistake—mishearing Robert Forte and starting things lower, at ten micrograms of LSD—has in the long run proved very beneficial.

Optimum Dose Level (LSD and Psilocybin)

What is the optimum dose level for LSD and psilocybin?

While this at first might seem like a reasonable question, it really isn't. It's the kind of question that makes sense if you're asking about pharmaceuticals, but not about microdoses.

One wouldn't, for example, ask someone about the optimum amount of string beans you should have with Thanksgiving dinner, or the optimum amount of Ben and Jerry's Phish Food ice cream you should have for dessert. It's easy to see not only that others can't decide for you but also that the answer depends on a whole host of variables that can change within you from meal to meal and, of course, vary even more from person to person. (There have to be people somewhere who don't like Phish Food, though we've never met any.)

The way to determine the right dose for you (at any time) is by *starting low, going slow, and regularly taking time off.* Ideally, your first dose will be too low, and you can gradually increase it until you're seeing some of the improvements being sought, yet you're not taking so much that its effects distract you.

The right dose for you? Start low. Go slow.

One benefit of working with a coach—simply because they have more experience—is they can help you zero in on the correct dose range or sweet spot sooner than you might on your own. In many cases people find they need less and less of a dose as they continue to microdose. It's not unusual after taking time off to find, when microdosing again, that they want less.

While your own awareness is the only sure guide to what's best for you, **the general recommended range of LSD (five to twelve micrograms) or psilocybin (one to three tenths of a gram of psilocybin-containing mushrooms) is right for most people,** but we have many reports of people successfully taking less, and there are some conditions where people need more to benefit. Also, psilocybin-containing mushrooms can be difficult to correctly dose because some species contain much greater concentrations of psilocybin[10] (as well as psilocin and baeocystin). You—and only you—can and must take full responsibility for determining your own best dose size.

Dose Levels for Other Substances

What about the other substances mentioned in this book, what is the right dosage for microdosing and what else should I know?

We won't—in many cases can't, and in other cases prefer not to—give you dose levels for microdosing all the substances mentioned in this book.

The **"can't"** refers to situations in which we can't specifically say, as we just don't know enough about it.

The **"won't"** refers to all the substances we classify as "Sometimes Spoken Of in Microdosing Terms" or "Not Recommended for Microdosing."

In addition to psilocybin and LSD, which have already been addressed, we're only going to discuss dosage for *B. caapi (Banisteriopsis caapi), Amanita muscaria,* and LSA. We will not be discussing a number of synthetics (like ALD-52 and 1p-LSD) similar to LSD.

A simple rule of thumb can help you determine a likely safe dose for any substance, natural or synthetic:

- A microdose is usually from one tenth to one twentieth of a full recreational dose, however that is calculated. To be safe, begin with a one twentieth amount or lower.
- If you find a trustworthy guide, teacher, shaman, or vendor, follow their instructions or start lower.
- Start very low and see what you feel; if there is a recommended dose level, start underneath it. Don't shy away from starting with just one drop of a tincture, regardless of its purported concentration and strength.

B. caapi: *Banisteriopsis caapi* is the scientific name for the yagé vine, also known as "soul vine." It's a giant South American liana (a long-stemmed woody vine) that grows up to thirty meters (almost a hundred feet) in length. It contains the alkaloids harmine, harmaline, and tetrahydroharmine.

B. caapi is most widely known as the major ingredient for the powerful psychedelic mixture ayahuasca, ceremonially used in many parts of South America for hundreds of years, and now used in contemporary rituals in many parts of the world. There are a number of religious organizations whose services center on the congregation's use of ayahuasca during the service. To make ayahuasca, *B. caapi* is boiled with any one of a number of plants containing DMT. The mixture allows the effects of the DMT to last for many hours.

The use of *B. caapi* as a microdose* is the central part of a complex protocol used by Microhuasca, a Peru-based organization that uses microdoses for healing. They developed a seven-week program and work with traditional ayahuasqueros and curanderos,† who individually

---

*The question often arises whether it is possible to successfully microdose using only the *B. caapi* vine—without an admixture of DMT coming in from another plant source. According to the Microhuasca organization: "Microdoses with only the ayahuasca vine (without DMT) show the same therapeutic effects as the conventional preparation of ayahuasca vine plus chacruna leaves. . . . According to qualitative reports, we have not found representative differentiation that can be attributed to the presence OR absence of DMT" (Microhuasca Institute, 2021).

†A "curandero" is a traditional South American indigenous healer, and an "ayahuasquero" is such a healer who specializes in working with ayahuasca.

prepare the medicine for each person in microdose quantities. During the program, individuals work with a guide and are also part of a mutual support group going through the process. In the week before taking their first dose, each group member navigates their own elements of care. This includes undertaking a *dieta* (a simplified healthy diet), setting intentions, and "fostering a conscious connection with the plant spirit."[11]

Each individual is then introduced to four levels of microdosing, from 5 percent of the ceremonial dose amount to 10, 15, and 20 percent. This allows individuals to discover the effects at each level and determine, with the help of their guide, their response at each level. From that point on, individuals decide what level of microdose to take on their dose day. Microdoses are taken following the Fadiman protocol, with each dose day being followed by two days without a dose. Throughout the following five weeks, each group member shares their experiences with the facilitators and other group members.

This microdosing program has been tried successfully with ayahuasca, San Pedro cactus, and psilocybin, as well as with psilocybin truffles (by the Microdosing Institute).

This is the first blended system, combining modern microdosing and traditional wisdom. Individuals interested in working this way should contact the program through Microhuasca.com. They have trained facilitators in ten countries and work with individuals in either Spanish or English.

A comprehensive guide to *B. caapi* and its use in microdosing is available online from the Microdosing Institute.[12]

***Amanita muscaria*:** Fly agaric, the red-and-white-flecked "Christmas" mushroom loved by Super Mario Bros., also known as *Amanita muscaria*, is not a classic psychedelic. Taken as a properly prepared microdose, however, it seems to have similar kinds of system-wide healing effects.

For those seriously interested in learning more about this mushroom, we suggest *Fly Agaric: A Compendium of History, Pharmacology, Mythology, and Exploration* (Feeney, 2020), and, for its physical and mental effects, *Microdosing with Amanita Muscaria* (Masha, 2022).

This mushroom grows near or under conifer and deciduous trees across much of North America, Europe, and Asia. It has been introduced into conifer forests in Australia and New Zealand as well and generally only grows wild. Commercial cultivation of *Amanita muscaria* has failed because of its complex symbiotic relationship with the roots of certain trees.

For microdosing, *Amanita muscaria* **must be correctly prepared** before it can be consumed safely; eating *Amanita muscaria* raw is a serious mistake.* The preparation process is called decarboxylation, and converts ibotenic acid into muscimol, the active psychedelic ingredient. Methods for decarboxylation are described online.

Warning: Do Not Consume Raw *Amanita Muscaria*

While this book does suggest that *Amanita muscaria* can be safe and effective, and in most places is a legal microdosing substance, it's absolutely, positively, indisputably true that eating or otherwise ingesting it in its raw form is not advisable, even at the microdose level.

Buying *Amanita muscaria* is legal in most countries. Baba Masha's book spurred numerous online offerings, not all of which were legitimate. Most people we've heard from who use *Amanita muscaria* for microdosing purposes take fully decarboxylated tinctures, prepared for low-dose and microdosing use.

---

*Most mushroom identification books label it as "toxic," which is true if it is not properly decarboxylated or taken at higher doses.

The dose range if you are using a tincture is 150 to 500 milligrams (half a gram). To be safest, start with one drop, and if you are not feeling or experiencing anything, move up slowly—ideally one drop at a time—until you find your sweet spot. Because higher doses have more dramatic effects, even the best tincture vendor may suggest a dose beyond the recommended microdose range. Fortunately, once you find your *Amanita muscaria* sweet spot, it is easy to dole out the correct number of drops.

LSA: "Acid's mild-mannered cousin, D-lysergic acid amide (LSA) . . . also known as ergine, is sometimes referred to as 'the natural LSD.'"[13] It is found in some morning glory seeds (*Rivea corymbosa, Ipomoea violacea*), with commercial names like "Heavenly Blue" and "Pearly Gates," as well as in Hawaiian baby woodrose seeds. These seeds are generally not very popular because of the nausea and fatigue often associated with taking them. To lessen the nausea, a tea or other liquid extraction can be made, and capsules with ground powder are also used.

Dose range: Of the two types of seeds, Hawaiian baby woodrose seeds have the higher concentration of LSA. For Hawaiian baby woodrose, use one seed or less for microdosing (making fractional parts of seeds that vary in potency can be tricky). For morning glory seeds, two to five seeds would be low, and up to twenty seeds would be at the high end. Always start low.

Optimal Dose Level Changes

Can someone's optimal dose level decrease (or increase) over time?

Yes, of course it can, simply because we as individuals change as our circumstances change over time.

For some people, the size of the microdose that lands them in the sweet spot is very stable and remains the same over time. Others find that over time (or from time to time) they have to reduce or (less commonly) increase their dose. If, for example, you feel you are starting to creep up and out of the microdosing zone on dosing days—if you experience any intoxication, psychedelic visuals, or noticeable alterations of normal consciousness—then you would want to lower your dose size.

Many factors are in play here, including how much stress someone is experiencing, how much sleep they are getting, and how healthy their gut and liver are. For example, higher gut and liver health leads to more psilocybin being converted into psilocin, so people who start eating better may need smaller doses. It may also be that as our minds and bodies "tune into" and experience what microdoses do with and for the body, we somehow become more efficient at doing so, necessitating a decreased dose. Alternatively, if we are facing new mental or physical health challenges, it may be that an increased dose is required to get into a new sweet spot.

Safe and effective microdosing requires ongoing attention and focus, as it requires a protocol, proper dosing, and regularly taking time off. Since dose levels can change as you change, it's something you always need to remain aware of.

Radically Smaller Doses

Do radically smaller doses than usual work for some people?

Some people successfully take amazingly low doses, down to one microgram of LSD or a hundredth of a gram of psilocybin-containing mushrooms.

A recent report said, "I took a tenth of a gram of psilocybin I'd measured myself, but it felt as if I had overdosed on coffee all day long." When she asked if microdosing might not be for her, it was suggested that she try taking half as much or less before she gave it up. She found that two hundredths of a gram lowered her anxiety and gave her greater focus in her work.

We don't have enough information to determine what kind of person does well on super-low doses, but often they describe themselves as being very sensitive to drugs, and usually take half or less of the dose of anything they're prescribed.

Early on, one person began microdosing in the hope that it might help her chronic migraines, as nothing else had provided any relief. She reported considerable success with ten micrograms of LSD. After about a month, she discovered that the physician who had made LSD capsules for her had made a mistake, and she'd actually been taking only one microgram. She elected to stay on that super-low dose.

Radically Higher Doses

What if I seem to need a lot more than the standard recommended microdose dose?

We sometimes get reports that say, "When I stay in the dose range you suggest, nothing happens, but when I double or sometimes triple that dose, I seem to have the same kinds of experiences that you report for people taking what you recommend." For some individuals in this category, taking psychedelics in these higher dose ranges seems to take away the veils and relax their ever-present social anxiety. As one report said:

> "I took forty mics before I went to the party, knowing full well I'd have my usual terrible time and end up withdrawn and be sorry I'd come. But miracle of miracles, I ended up talking with almost everyone, and they seemed to want to stay in conversation with me. When the party ended, I was desperate to find someone else to talk to while I was in this state. I drove around until I found a bar that was open late and went in and talked with people until it closed. It was as if I'd lived my life in black and white and, for the first time, I could see color."

In almost every case, the person identified as, or was similar to, people who are high-functioning on the autism scale. See our later discussion of these neurodivergent individuals—with their advantages and challenges—and how they use higher doses almost exactly like people who take doses in the normal range.

Adjusting for Body Weight

Should a bigger person take a bigger dose? (I weigh three hundred pounds.)

No, it is not a good idea to adjust the dose for microdosing based on body weight.

In 2021, Albert Garcia-Romeu et al. published a study titled "Optimal dosing for psilocybin pharmacotherapy: Considering weight-adjusted and fixed dosing approaches." They concluded that "across a wide range of body weights (49 to 113 kg) the present results showed no evidence that body weight affected the subjective effects of psilocybin."[14]

While this study looked only at high-dose psilocybin use, there's no evidence to suggest that body weight–adjusted doses make a beneficial difference for microdosing with any substance.

Any adjustment away from the recommended dose range for the substance you are using should be entirely based on personal, individual experience. As discussed throughout, going slow and starting low always makes the most sense, as does testing out your proposed dose range on a day where you don't have to go anywhere or have any scheduled commitments.

Variability of Dose Levels

Do some physical or mental medical conditions require different dose levels than the ones described above?

People used to microdosing, and who are having difficult symptoms or feel no change in their underlying condition, will often ask if a higher dose would be better. Usually, it's the other way around—it's a lower dose that will be more effective. That is, for nearly every

health condition we've seen, the general trend is that instead of someone maintaining or increasing their dose level, less and less over time is
likely to be more effective.

Wanting to Up the Dose

***I find myself wanting to take more–a bigger dose–to keep feeling or
even intensify the effects. Mo' betta, right?***

With microdosing, *less is more*. When starting, take enough time,
focus, and patience to begin with a low dose level and ratchet it up
until it's just a *little* too much—then back off just one notch. That
will enable you to stay at a best-for-now dose for you—no substantial
changes of ordinary consciousness, no intoxication, no trouble in getting through your regular day.

Suppose everything is going well, but at some point, you find yourself wondering about raising the dose—perhaps just a wee bit.

"If some is good, then more is better." When something is good or
wonderful, we may sometimes want more and more of it. That's rarely
the right decision, but the desire is real. Controlling the "more-mores"*—
whether for Phish Food or our personal favorite hedonistic activity—is
something that most of us have had to learn how to do or are still working on.

Jim and Jordan's book (*Your Symphony of Selves,* 2020) describes
how all of us have different selves or parts, each of which can have different interests, needs, and feelings—all of which need to be respected.
However, some of our parts can act out or create problems.

Why might part of you suggest having a bit more "just to see"?

Perhaps some prior symptoms are coming back. Maybe you are
looking to reignite the same creative zing that showed up when you
first tried microdosing. Or perhaps part of you believes you're no longer
at the optimal dose, and that it's time to experiment.

---

*This wonderful phrase and idea comes from Avi Esther, Natural Medicine Woman.

Either you decide to follow the impulse to raise your dose and see what happens, or you don't.

If you experiment, do it sensibly. Raise the dose level just a little, and do it on a day where you're in a safe place, so that if it turns out to be too much, things will still be okay. Then evaluate whether what you're experiencing works for you.*

The most common reason admitted to by people who want more is the hope that a higher dose will provide a little bit of the flavor of psychedelic consciousness change—both pleasurable and perhaps just at the edge of being distracting. That's *not* the ideal microdosing dose. However, if your underlying symptoms have improved, or your physical agility or creative productivity has increased, or you find yourself more comfortable in social situations, you may want to stay at or at least occasionally visit this higher dose.

You're always the only person who can correctly calibrate your own use. Remember, though, that if you frequently find yourself pushing your own limits—if you give in too much or too often to the more-mores— then you'll likely end up experiencing less-less of the potential benefits that working with microdosing can bring.

Overdose Potential

Even if you're just microdosing, is it possible to overdose and get into trouble?

Reddit's r/microdosing subreddit had a report from an individual who, after two months of successful microdosing, said he had a monthlong psychotic episode. His dose was .33 grams of psilocybin-containing mushrooms embedded in chocolate, four days on, three days

---

*Carefully follow your dosing protocol, especially if raising your dose. Consider this report: "I've done lots of full trips, so didn't worry about raising my microdose. I ended up in an unscheduled meeting, and was phasing in and out of being there. I got a note that said, 'Are you high? You're making no sense.' I stood up, muttered 'Don't feel well,' and got out of there. Almost cost me my job."

Moral: Raise your dose on your own time.

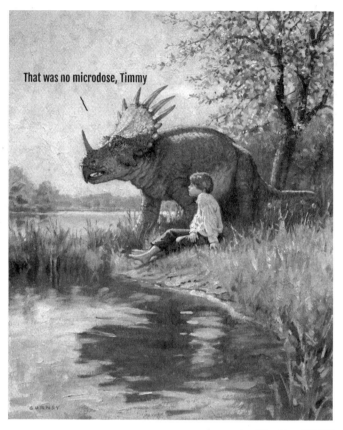

Image © James Gurney, BDSP, 2006

off. Except being told that "the shrooms were helping me in a lot of ways (productivity, mood, confidence, etc.),"[15] we know very little else about what happened. The remarkably sophisticated r/microdosing community had no explanation beyond the possibility of an overdose, since "psilocybin sometimes blends very unevenly into chocolate."[16]

In high-dose sessions, where an overdose is always possible, people are counseled to seek a quiet place with someone to stay with them for the few hours it takes for the high dose to wear off.

While it's more difficult to overdose with microdoses, it certainly can happen. Taking psychological shelter in place with a trusted person and avoiding unnecessary medical interventions can leave enough time for things to resolve on their own. (We know of situations where insufficiently trained medical or legal personnel overreacted, making things much worse and causing lasting negative impacts.) So while we know of situations where high-dose overdoses have been problematic, we aren't aware of any microdosing-related overdoses that caused any trouble.

Verifying Dose and Substance

Can I verify what I'm taking is really the substance and dose it's supposed to be?

If you're not sure if what you've bought is the substance you intended, test it to be safe and sure. Dangerous substances have been sold as LSD, like 2C-I-NBOMe, and recently, with the sudden popularity of *Amanita muscaria,* there has been a rise in online stores claiming they are selling you *Amanita muscaria* (often as gummies), when that's not necessarily what you receive.

Test kits are available online from DanceSafe.org, Amazon.com, and other sources. We learned from James McConchie, proprietor of the Haight Street Shroom Shoppe, that a test-at-home kit for psilocybin potency—the "Psilocybin QTest"—has recently come to market; it's described as "the world's first and only potency test kit for accurately measuring psilocybin contents from magic mushrooms."[17]

Properly prepared microdoses are physically safe for almost everyone. You need to know with a reasonable degree of certainty that what you intend to ingest satisfies two criteria:

- It is the desired substance or combination of substances and nothing else.
- The dose level of the substance(s) is as advertised.

If you're growing your own psilocybin mushrooms, or picking and properly preparing your own *Amanita muscaria,* or growing San Pedro cactus, you will have the ultimate trusted source: yourself. You will need a digital scale that goes down to 0.01 grams (available on Amazon.com).

If you have a trusted friend or family member who shares with you what they have used or their source, you're in good hands. If, however, you don't have any direct connection to your final source—no personal vouchsafing or recommendation—then **test the substance.** A safety-first approach necessarily includes a test-at-home kit.

If something doesn't look, feel, or smell right, or your intuition tells you something is amiss, then stop. *Better safe than sorry.* Go about finding or creating a source you feel better about.

One of the benefits of the increasing legalization of psychedelics throughout the world will be accurately labeled substances for microdosing and macrodosing. A 2023 law review article puts it this way: "One of the greatest potential benefits of legalizing and regulating psychedelics . . . is the availability of accurate and consistent doses that are correctly labeled, unadulterated with other substances, and uncontaminated by pesticides and other toxins. . . . Psychedelic substances obtained from illicit sources may have variable and unpredictable potency."[18]

We can look forward to brand-name microdosing products—as discussed in "Predictions" on page 278—but in the meantime, be as safe as you can by taking all necessary precautions.

Protocols: Keeping to a Schedule and Taking Breaks

What are the different microdosing "protocols" or schedules?

The word "protocol" simply means "schedule," or how often—and for how long—one should microdose. All protocols are variations of the same basic rule:

✦ **Start low, go slow, and take time off.**
   Or this version:
✦ **Not too much, not too often, and not too long without a break.**

I like day two the best. So calm, and so much control
over my emotions and reactions!
—ER nurse

Day two is better.
—CEO of multinational corporation

Protocols in widespread use include:[19]

- **Fadiman Protocol:** Dose on day one, no dose on days two and three. Dose on day four, no dose on days five and six. And so on.
- **Stamets Protocol:** Dose for 4 days in a row, then take 3 days with no dose.
- **Microdosing Institute Protocol:** Every other day until you take time off.
- **Nightcap Protocol:** Take a microdose before going to sleep, otherwise following one of the above protocols.
- **Intuitive Protocol:** People with enough experience base their microdosing schedules on prior results and intuition. The general rules above as to time off and breaks still apply. Keep in mind that the lower dose level is the preferred decision.
- *Amanita muscaria* **Protocols:**
  » *Baba Masha:* Take morning and evening, unless insomnia results, then take morning dose only. Take doses every day for three weeks. Stop for four to seven days to observe changes. Repeat three-week course and then take another break. Effects are cumulative. No more than four or five courses a year. (Masha, 2022)
  » *All Things Amanita:* This website (allthingsamanita.com) recommends the Fadiman and Stamets protocols.

Note that all the protocols but Masha's for *Amanita muscaria* include days off to prevent tolerance—needing more of a substance to get the same or possibly no effect—and all the protocols include longer breaks on a regular basis.

If you are microdosing for the first time—and aren't working with or haven't worked with a coach, program, or class—it is prudent to dose with one of the above tested and validated protocols, within the recommended dose range. Having an easy-to-follow structure like this lets you focus on what you're noticing, your intention setting, ongoing integration, and so on.

Time off: Remember that all these protocols include taking two or so weeks off after every four to six weeks on a protocol.

Differences Among Protocols

What are the differences among protocols?

While the dose level information in this book is pooled from a number of sources, there has been no research to date comparing the effectiveness of one protocol over another for any specific condition. There were different reasons for the creation of the Fadiman protocol, the Stamets protocol, the every-other-day protocol, the "intuitive" protocol, the "nightcap" protocol, and others. Each has its advocates, but ultimately individual users determine what works best for them.

People microdosing for the first time often ask, "I'm not sure it's working. Would it be better for me to take it more often?" The answer is usually "stay where you started for a few weeks; then review it." Usually, after a few weeks, people find whatever protocol they're on to be satisfactory. If not, they may microdose more or less often. Paul Stamets said it best: "One can't be too rigid."

(A few conditions, like pain from shingles, have special protocols, which are described later, in chapter 5.)

Second-Day Effect

What is it? You can barely find online references to it.

The Fadiman protocol is to dose on day one, not dose on days two and three, then dose on day four . . . and repeat for up to six weeks, then take a couple of weeks off.

Following some initial reports of positive effects being experienced on the second day, Jim asked additional early participants to take a second day off. That is, as he continued to explore how microdosing affected people, Jim asked them to not dose again until the third day after dosing to give them time to return to baseline before re-dosing. The second-day effect was an unanticipated discovery, but is now reflected in many microdosing protocols and in a number of research studies.

Two years later, at a Wisconsin conference, Jim was having dinner with Johns Hopkins professor Roland Griffiths, who was skeptical of any second-day effect. At that moment, "Edward," whose company had sponsored the conference, walked by. He paused and said to Jim, "The second day is really the best." Roland was impressed by the synchronicity. Johns Hopkins, however, has yet to approve a microdosing study.

To date, no formal studies have been done on the second-day effect or how common it is. However, all the protocols (except some for *Amanita muscaria*) include days off. This is in sharp distinction from most pharmaceuticals, which are taken daily or even more often.

While we now describe the advantages of taking days off in terms of increasing safety and decreasing potential undesired effects, it came into being for entirely different reasons.

Taking Just One Microdose

Are there benefits from trying microdosing just once?

In the world of high-dose psychedelics, there are many instances where even a single dose of a psychedelic can cause long-lasting positive effects and outcomes. It is not unusual, for example, for scientific studies to give individuals just one macrodose. We know from research on neuroplasticity that even one high dose of psychedelics can improve health for a month or longer.

With microdosing, however, as we are dealing with much smaller doses, while it is possible that a single microdose may have positive effects, it is much less likely. Microdosing relies on the *cumulative effects* of taking small doses on a regular schedule. If you take just one dose, it is unlikely you will experience very much on the dose day or on the following days. Put differently, *taking one microdose is not really microdosing,* so you can't expect the known benefits of microdosing to follow.

Every Day

Most prescription medications are taken every day, and ones for mental health, like SSRIs, are taken daily for years. We take our daily vitamins, so why not our daily microdoses? If microdosing really is inherently safe, would it hurt anything?

The obvious answer is: "No!" Psychedelics are *not* like prescription medications and are not taken like daily vitamins.

As already noted, all protocols described in this book include taking days off and time off—often considerable time off. All protocols but one (*Amanita muscaria*) include days off during active dosing.

The first protocol explored, the Fadiman protocol—one day of dosing and two days without—was designed to take advantage of an early finding that, for many people, a single dose lasted two days; people were still feeling better, seeing things more clearly, etc., on the second day. As a practical matter, if something lasts for two days, it is pointless and wasteful to take it more often.

There is ample evidence that macrodoses of psychedelics lose effectiveness within a few days if taken daily. All groups who have independently established organizations for microdosing coaching, support, or simply sales recommend taking days off and then, following finishing a protocol, taking a longer break that lasts for some weeks.

We have no evidence that microdosing on a daily basis is beneficial. On the other hand, we do have reports like the following, from a science writer with more than ten years of microdosing experience, someone who has tried many variations with many substances:

> "If I microdose every day, it doesn't work as well. I'm not as clear. Even if I do go every other day for a while, I make sure to take off at least a couple of days after not very long."

We have a few reports from people on the Stamets protocol (four days on, then three days off) reporting negative experiences that resolved when they went to a protocol with a day or more between each dose.

There are no benefits reported from microdosing every day. Don't do it.

Taking Time Off

I've been coached to microdose for six weeks and then take a few weeks off. Why is this important, and what's going on during this time?

All suggested protocols today (except for *Amanita muscaria*) include days off during each week of microdosing, and all advise taking some weeks off after several weeks of weekly dosing.*

At this point, taking time off may seem like settled science. But how the days and weeks off came into being had nothing to do with science or medicine, and nothing to do with thousands of years of indigenous use.

Acting independently, individuals and groups across the United States, Holland, and even South America—using entirely different substances—decided that taking a few weeks off was a healthy idea. No research, science, or even any theory—and certainly no data—was responsible for this independently generated consensus. While there

---

*A good rule of thumb is to take off no more than half the number of weeks you microdosed. Four weeks of microdosing means no more than two weeks off. Six weeks equals no more than three weeks off.

is no university, research organization, independent clinical group, or anyone else testing the difference between taking time off and not taking time off, the practice is nearly universally agreed upon.

It is beneficial to sometimes allow one's system to work on its own. This prevents dependence and adds to microdosing's safety profile. And taking time off between a series of doses makes any health concerns less likely.

Taking a break gives you time to reflect on and integrate your experience. You can determine how microdosing is working for you, and may want to adjust your protocol, either in terms of dosing days or dose level. If you have access to more than one microdosing substance, you might want to try something else, but if you are pleased with your results so far, you've no need to experiment. You may also feel that you have achieved the results you hoped for and stop entirely.

Reports suggest that by taking a break, you will enjoy, appreciate, and recognize what has worked or not worked for you. Should you resume microdosing at any time following a break, you will be better informed and more aware of why you are doing so and how best to take advantage of it.

Contraindications, Safety Concerns, and Other Cautions

Side Effects

What are the side effects of microdosing LSD? Psilocybin? Other substances?

A useful answer here takes some explanation: **there are no side effects to any of these substances.** There are also no side effects to alcohol, coffee, aspirin, antidepressants, cannabis, and so on.

The term "side effects" is a universally accepted way of describing the undesirable effects of a medication or procedure. It is also one of the most remarkable yet unacknowledged advertising scams of the century, a brilliant marketing term that we all have come to associate with the usually minor and undesirable effects of a medication.

Important: Half Then Half Again

Almost all reported negative effects of microdosing can be eliminated by lowering the dose, starting by cutting it in half. If the undesired effects persist, cut it in half once more. If the problem STILL persists, then **stop microdosing**, as it is not right for you at this time. Nothing is good for everybody, and some things are good for us only at certain points in our lives.

A more useful approach is to recognize that there are *desired* effects, *most likely* effects, *rare* effects, *unpleasant* effects, *dangerous* effects, and so on. Once you shake your mind loose of the notion that the advertised effect is the primary or real effect and all other effects are somehow minor or just "side" portions, everything you experience makes more sense.

Nearly any substance can have one or more undesirable effects. People die every year from internal bleeding caused by aspirin. Tylenol can damage the liver; a harmful dose is close enough to a therapeutic dose that this fact is mentioned on the bottle. Antidepressants have numerous negative effects, and many people who smoke cannabis experience paranoia. Regardless of what the marketing or medical people would have you believe, for those experiencing them, these effects can be the main course—not on the side at all.

Classic psychedelics in general, even in high doses, are physiologically among the safest drugs we know of. Microdoses are even safer. However, there is an ongoing question as to whether some people who microdose over long periods of time may experience cumulative negative effects.

Immediate uncomfortable effects of a microdosing experience may include heightened anxiety, headaches, tinnitus, or sleep disturbances. Psilocybin-containing mushrooms can cause brief bouts of nausea. Almost all the reports in our database show that for most people, uncomfortable effects are alleviated by taking a reduced dose, or taking doses less often. If undesired effects continue, people usually just stop microdosing.

Published research agrees that microdosing has a remarkably good safety track record, although larger surveys have uncovered a wide range of potential negative effects. A 2020 review article by Ona and Bouso[20] described categories of potential negative effects on mood, including increased anxiety, sadness, irritability, and symptoms of depression. The article also mentions the potential for:

- **Physical discomfort:** overstimulation, disrupted senses, and temperature dysregulation.
- **Adverse events related to cognitive functioning:** distractibility, absentmindedness, and decreased performance on cognitive tasks.
- **Mental health issues:** insomnia, dissociation, depersonalization, rumination, and overanalysis.
- **Impaired social skills:** awkwardness, oversharing, difficulties with sentence production.

The most common unwanted effects reported were anxiety and insomnia. Unfortunately, few of the studies looked at in this meta-study included specific percentages or numbers of individuals who had any of these negative effects.

What we have learned is that the majority of negative symptoms—most of them quite rare—are linked to taking too large a dose, and in some cases, to a bad current life situation. The most common undesirable microdosing effect comes *from taking too large a dose and feeling a little bit high.* If that occurs, it's best to treat the experience as you would treat an even higher dose: stay where you are, if possible, and be quiet, listen to music, or spend the time in nature, or with friends or pets, until the effects diminish.

An example reported to us came from someone working in sales, who had been microdosing successfully and valuing the results. However, one day, he decided that if ten micrograms were good, twenty would probably be wonderful. After taking that dose, he went to his workplace and attended an important sales meeting. As he listened, he recognized that he really had no interest in the product. A short time later, he had the additional realization that he also had no interest in sales. Wisely, at that point, he left the meeting and returned home. He said he did not make that mistake again.

Psychotic Episodes

Can microdosing trigger a psychotic episode?

While rare events do happen, at least as far as we know—with tens of thousands of individuals over the past ten years reporting their microdosing experiences—there have been no reports of psychotic episodes having been triggered by microdosing.

So why are there warnings like this one, which comes from an article on microdosing on Harvard University's "Science in the News" webpage?

> The question, however, is not just whether microdosing is effective, but also whether it's safe. Until clinical trials are complete, we will not have a full answer, but there is already research to suggest that certain people may be vulnerable to negative side effects. In particular, some people may have psychotic episodes or other mental health issues triggered by taking psychedelics, especially if they have a history of psychosis or pre-existing risk for serious psychiatric disorders

like schizophrenia or bipolar disorder. Although microdosing involves a much lower amount of the drug, it is still possible that the negative consequences may hold true.[21]

While almost anything is "still possible," we are not sure that clinical trials will ever be sufficiently "complete" such that we'll "have a full answer."

If anything, the research seems to suggest there is little cause for concern. Consider the title and subtitle of a 2015 *Scientific American* article on high doses: "No Link Found Between Psychedelics and Psychosis—A large US survey found that users of LSD and similar drugs were no more likely to have mental-health conditions than other respondents."[22] Similarly, Dana Smith's 2023 *New York Times* article, "Psychedelics Are a Promising Therapy, but They Can Be Dangerous for Some," tells us the following:

> What little data does exist suggests that the chances of psychosis developing in the general population is low. One survey of over 1,000 self-reporting recreational psychedelic users did not find a link between drug use and schizophrenia-like symptoms. Another study similarly showed no connection between past psychedelic use and current psychosis or other psychiatric disorders.[23]

Still, people with a prior history of psychosis might wish to consult with a knowledgeable professional before considering microdosing.

Taking Too Much by Mistake

Is it easy to mess up and take more than a microdose? Are there safeguards?

When individuals with no previous psychedelic experience decide to microdose, they rarely make this mistake. It is not uncommon, however, for psychonauts with considerable psychedelic experience to be more lax and casual about their dosing and occasionally have problems.

Mistakes happen. A friend received a gift in the mail from another friend who knew he was microdosing. There were some tabs of paper infused with LSD, and a note commenting about the value of microdosing. Pleased with the gift, and without asking his friend, *he assumed that each tab was a microdose,* as has been becoming more common in the psychedelic underground.

A few days later, finishing up some morning work, he took one tab and prepared to go to lunch with some former students. Cognitively, he felt fine, but he soon realized that what he'd taken seemed like a strong microdose. He asked his wife to join him and do the driving. At the restaurant, when their order arrived, he looked down at the food, and, when it looked back at him, he realized what must have happened. Looking into the brightly illuminated faces of his friends, and failing to explain what had happened, he asked his wife to take him home. He spent the afternoon lying quietly on the couch, his dog snuggled up beside him. He had actually taken the one hundred micrograms that were in that single tab.

There are ways of bringing people down from high doses (such as using benzodiazepines and niacin), but they are not recommended. The staff at the Zendo Project, who help overdosed individuals at Burning Man and other festivals, say, "We don't bring people down, we do bring them through" (so they can complete their experience, but in a safe space).

The best and ideal safeguard, of course, is to know what and how much you're taking—and then double-check both. If there's any concern whatsoever, don't guess, but instead wait for another day when you can be sure that you're dosing yourself correctly.

There's a story from the Sufi tradition (a religious order within Islam) attributed to Jesus. Seen running from a village, Jesus was asked by a believer what could have possibly frightened him. Jesus paused and said, "I can raise the dead, but I cannot help the stupid" . . . and continued to run.

Mistakes happen. People drop cell phones off bridges, lose their car keys, break favorite dishes, forget to pay their light bills, and mis-dose psychedelics. There are valuable lessons to be learned from mistakes. However, it's usually better not to have to learn those lessons by personal experience. Better to learn by observing others than to be the one others learn from.

Contraindicated Medications and Conditions

What medication and psychological and physical conditions are contraindicated with microdosing? Any authoritative resources?

There are many different medications and treatments for the world's physical and mental conditions. We know of no authoritative list or final arbiter of which among them is contraindicated for microdosing.

What we offer, however, is a list of medications, supplements, and herbs that have been reported as being safe to take while microdosing. See the appendix (page 299) for the most current list at publication.[24] Additional entries will be made to the list as they are reported.

Long-Term Safety and Impact

Is there any research on the long-term safety and impact of microdosing on human beings?

Long-term studies on almost *any* pharmaceutical are undertaken far less often than one might think. Drugs like SSRIs, for example, are rarely studied for as long as a full year, even though individuals take them for decades (Kirsch, 2010). Such studies are enormously expensive, and there is very little upside for the original manufacturer to undertake them, as even the most profitable drug eventually gives way to a far less expensive generic equivalent.

The US federal government did a couple of long-range studies on long-term use of antidepressants, comparing individuals in the drug-prescribed group with those in a control group with a similar diagnosis over a twenty-year period. The studies determined that people who *had not taken medication* for their mental conditions did better in the long run than those who had been medicated.[25]

Alternatively, there have been studies digging into massive government records, contrasting those who took psychedelics (almost all high doses) and those who did not. One study found that people who had taken psychedelics were physically healthier; another, looking only at individuals who had been incarcerated, showed that those with psychedelics in their backgrounds committed fewer violent crimes than those who had never used psychedelics.

Jim knows people who have microdosed for more than two decades. They seem physically and psychologically healthy, although they may have been that way before their first psychedelic journeys. There has been some speculation, which we cover elsewhere, about potential physical damage among long-term users, both macrodosers and micro-dosers. No evidence has yet been found for long-term physical damage caused by the classic psychedelics (LSD, psilocybin, mescaline, DMT).

Another place we looked for relevant information is among indigenous users. To date, we have no reports of groups changing their use pattern or altogether stopping the traditional use of high or low doses of the fungi and plants available to them.

If we think of microdosing the way we think of vitamins, we become less concerned with negative long-term effects and more interested in determining if the desired effects are maintained over time. That is, the focus turns to working more effectively with what microdosing makes possible.

Best Practices, Guidance, and Outside Assistance

Sourcing Psychedelics

What are the safest and best ways and places to find sources of psychedelics to microdose?

We can't help you here.

The situation differs in every country and is constantly changing. We have described how various rules about psychedelics in general—and psilocybin in particular—differ from country to country and, at least in the United States, from state to state. In some countries specific psychedelics are legal, in others legal with restrictions, in still others illegal on paper but not enforced against, and in some countries illegal with some enforcement. For example, *Amanita muscaria* is currently legal in all US states except Louisiana, and in most other countries with notable exceptions including Australia, the Netherlands, Romania, Thailand, and possibly Great Britain.

In jurisdiction after jurisdiction, laws are shifting toward greater availability. Remember: it was a political—not a medical or scientific—decision by the Nixon administration to restrict the availability of these substances in the first place and to pressure other countries to follow suit. Now, with individual use and medical and clinical research expanding, and with commercial companies approaching being able to sell their products, restrictions are being rolled back throughout the world. Check your local and national laws to determine what specific restrictions remain.

When friends, colleagues, or online strangers ask us to help with sourcing, we suggest they look to local groups, or to individuals they know who are already interested in or more experienced with psychedelics, or to commercial companies selling reliable mushroom grow kits.*

---

*In 1976, Terence and Dennis McKenna published their *Psilocybin: Magic Mushroom Grower's Guide,* which

As things stand now, the US Drug Enforcement Agency (DEA) has confirmed the *legality* of the spores themselves: "If the mushroom spores (or any other material) do not contain psilocybin or psilocin (or any other controlled substance or listed chemical), the material is considered not controlled."[26]

Over five years ago, we received requests from more than fifty-one countries asking how to best use psychedelics for microdosing. As our website then said, "*Don't ask us about sources,*" these requests were all from people who had already found a way to solve their own sourcing needs.

As of mid-2024, there seems to be a rush of online companies selling microdoses (and more) as if there were no legal concerns. Some are in Canada; some are touted by influencers on TikTok and elsewhere. It was not always like this.

For Ayelet Waldman, the author of 2017's bestselling *A Really Good Day: How Microdosing Made a Mega Difference in My Mood, My Marriage, and My Life,* finding a source wasn't easy. As a successful attorney, author, and lecturer, Ayelet found that conventional medications were not helping with her mental illness. After coming across *The Psychedelic Explorer's Guide* (Fadiman, 2011) and then consulting with Jim, she decided to try microdosing.

In her book, she described how difficult it was, even in Berkeley, for a straight middle-aged person to find a source of illegal psychedelics. By following up on her friendships with faculty in different departments throughout UC Berkeley, by openly expressing her concerns and desires, and by following through despite several fumbles and failures, she eventually received some LSD in the mail from an elderly professor who said he was not likely to use it this lifetime. This was in 2015.

It's easier now to find microdoses than it was for Ayelet. In part, the favorable coverage of the benefits of psychedelics in general in the

---

laid out a reliable method for growing mushrooms at home. Since then, with accumulated know-how and technical advances, it has become much simpler. Today's one-stop kits come with everything you need but the spores.

past few years, and of microdosing in particular, has led to enhanced availability.

In early 2024, there were articles in *The Wall Street Journal*[27] and *The Times* (London)[28] describing how a number of professional women in each country easily and regularly use microdosing to improve their busy lives. Neither article mentioned any difficulty in sourcing. As we were writing this segment, Jim was shown an iridescent packet of "PsycheJellies—Choose Your Own Adventure" gummies, each one containing a tenth of a gram of psilocybin mushrooms.* A week later, he was offered a small bright yellow plastic tube containing forty tiny tablets, each one 0.25 grams. On the side of the tube was written: "Happiness Tabs."

Jordan confirms that for the people he knows, having increasing access to preprepared psilocybin capsules, usually in .125 and .25 doses, has changed the game in terms of ease of use. As a friend of his put it, "Not only do you no longer have to store, cut, and weigh whole mushrooms, but you don't have to expend any particular preparation time or energy at the start of a dose day. It's very convenient; ready for you, when you're ready for it."

> The times they are a-changin'.
> —Bob Dylan

Mixing High and Low Doses

I really like how microdosing treats me. But I want to go deeper, maybe take a full dose. I have friends who do both, off and on.

We all tend to suffer from the same mindset, thinking that a big amount of something has essentially the same but stronger effects than a small amount. This is true in lots of cases. Until a shift happens.

---

*Jim's friend told him that he got them from a woman he only knows from church, who told him she orders it from "somewhere."

A couple of aspirin does more for reducing inflammation or pain than a single aspirin, but adding aspirin onto aspirin at some point leads to internal bleeding. The ibuprofen label says that if you take more than a certain amount per day, it can cause liver damage. One drink makes you more cheerful and more social, and four might make you think you're more sexy and clever. A few more? You can't stand upright, and you can barely make it to the toilet before you throw up.

There's a world of information out there on how to benefit from high doses. Jim's book *The Psychedelic Explorer's Guide* is one of the popular ones. There is no lack of wonderful descriptive books, from Aldous Huxley's to Michael Pollan's, as well as personal sagas, adventures with indigenous teachers, advice from shamans, memoirs, and idiosyncratic revelations. Online classes, meetups, retreats, one-on-one individual trainings, and lots more are available, all geared to safe and beneficial high-dose sessions.

None of the high-dose effects focused on in these books, resources, or other opportunities are relevant to microdosing. High doses affect the body-mind-spirit with different beneficial effects, different potential negative effects, and a whole raft of effects that will never be experienced by anyone microdosing. While so much is available about maximizing the potential of higher doses, none of that—repeat, none of that—directly relates to microdosing. Macrodosing and microdosing are each most effective when properly practiced in their own domain.

One piece of advice we can give is that using high doses or microdoses without taking sufficient time between them lowers their effectiveness. Therefore, if you want to take a high dose, it's best to stop microdosing for a week or two before. And you may not find any value in returning to microdosing for anywhere from several days to a few weeks thereafter.

Finally, if you are returning to microdosing after a high dose, consider starting with a smaller dose than you previously used. People sometimes find they've been "tuned up" by their high-dose experience so that a smaller-sized microdose becomes better for finding and staying in the sweet spot.

Trauma-Informed Practitioner

I'm deciding between a couple of microdosing coaches, and one says she's "trauma informed." What does that mean, and is it important?

A hot topic in the worlds of therapy, coaching, and self-help psychology is *trauma*—what it is, how it gets stored or "locked into" the body's tissues and neural wiring, how it impacts us, and what to do to release it. Popular books,[29] podcasts, and courses by medical providers, coaches, and therapists focus on how to effectively work with and heal trauma and its impacts without further "triggering" or re-stimulating the trauma.

There isn't widespread agreement as to exactly what a trauma-informed approach consists of, despite a host of certification programs. Trauma-informed therapy has a mind-body-spirit orientation in recognizing and addressing the long-lasting impacts of adverse events. It draws from the insights of humanistic and transpersonal psychology and includes practices from many healing schools and modalities, including somatic and body-based therapies (massage, therapeutic healing touch, yoga, breathwork, meditation, progressive muscle relaxation), expressive arts methods (art therapy, music therapy, writing, dancing, singing), group, companion, and animal therapy, and more.

Trauma-informed professionals understand *the importance of safety* in achieving positive outcomes. You can't and won't heal—even with the resources to do so—unless you feel safe.[30] They work with clients to create and maintain internal feelings of safety regardless of what's happening or what comes up.

What, then, about the extra effort and possibly expense needed to find and work with someone who is trauma informed? There's a much, much smaller likelihood of being triggered into a traumatized self and into physically or emotionally reliving the trauma and its pain when microdosing than when working with high doses.

However, the trauma-informed approach has revealed that there doesn't have to be a single large traumatic event in someone's life for them to suffer from trauma. Small repeated traumas—a thousand little cuts from physical or emotional events that are distressing and cause pain or otherwise make us unhappy—can leave us with dysfunctional attributes.*

If you feel that you may find yourself "in" or being directly affected by a traumatized part of who you are, and you have decided to work with a microdosing professional, it may indeed make sense to seek out someone who is "trauma informed."

Microdosing and Psychotherapy

Now that I'm microdosing and feeling so much better, is it better to continue with or drop my weekly psychotherapy session?

Begin by talking things over with your therapist, just as you would (or should) do if you were considering discontinuing therapy for any other reason.

From reviewing reports from individuals who had the same decision to make and decided to stay with their therapist, and from talking with therapists with clients who are microdosing, it appears that microdosers make better use of therapy than they did previously. They are better able to stay present and go deeper with difficult or disturbing memories or habit patterns, and they are able to better use the insights and tools learned during the course of therapy. Clients often say that while prior to microdosing they understood the value of these tools, they weren't as able (or maybe as willing) to make use of them.

Stay in therapy until therapy stops being useful. Fortunately, microdosing improves the effectiveness of therapy.

---

*Microdosing may give you more awareness of your different selves and how they interact, but it can also intensify the feelings and pains of a given self. Microdosing provides a window of opportunity that allows you to form new neural connections and pathways or to let go of old dysfunctional ones.

Recommendations for Coaches, Retreats, Groups

I'm just getting started; who or what groups do you recommend?

This is not an easy question, for a few reasons.

It used to be difficult to not be able to help people. When asked, what we now suggest is this: "*Ask your friends, google the word 'psychedelic' and where you're living. Find out if there is an interest group near you. If there is, we recommend you attend a meeting and let people there know of your interests.*" We have been amazed how often, within just a few days, we'll get an email back such as: "Thanks! I've made a connection."

The purpose of this book is to give you as much information as we can so that you can make more informed decisions for yourself. We are not and cannot be a personal referral service.

Additional Considerations

Are there other things—besides substance, dose, how often to take it, and when to take time off—that I should think about before starting microdosing?

There are a number of additional considerations worth looking at, including set and setting, integration, "regular day," minimum duration, and working with others, some of which have already been covered in part in "Protocols: Keeping to a Schedule and Taking Breaks," on page 58.

SET AND SETTING

Do "set and setting" guidelines for taking large doses of psychedelics also apply to microdosing?

We've spoken a good deal about correct dose size, but haven't emphasized "set and setting."

"Set" refers to your intentions and expectations—your "mindset"— whenever you take any size dose of any psychedelic. "Setting" refers to your physical, social, and cultural environment—the room, the people you are with, and your current life situation.

"Set and setting" is not as crucial with microdosing as it is with high doses, but it still helps to anchor or improve microdosing as well.

For example, if you feel angry, disoriented, or unsupported, you may want to wait until you're on a more even keel before beginning a microdosing protocol. If things are going very wrong in your external life, it may be better to wait until your life settles down before starting microdosing. Knowing why you are microdosing and paying special attention to that particular aspect of your life or health will likely yield better results than just microdosing and hoping for the best. Focused expectancy is useful in achieving goals in general.

In the end, it is more about how you feel about the setting than the setting itself.

INTEGRATION

Integration is one of those buzzwords that seems to be everywhere. Is it really something you have to do, and do you have to work with a coach to do it?

"Integration" means taking stock of what you experience while incorporating new realizations and behaviors into your life. While following a protocol, you become aware of and can fine-tune the changes you're experiencing. For example, if microdosing helps you feel less anxious and gives you more energy, taking time to reflect on this can help you continue your progress. Integration does not require anyone else's participation.

REGULAR DAY

Will there be any problem in having my regular day?

If you are taking the correct dose, you won't experience any disorientating psychedelic effects. Therefore, there's no reason why anything that comes up should be a problem. If something completely unexpected comes up, you might feel things a bit more intensely, but if anything, you might find yourself more grounded, centered, and resourceful.

MINIMUM DURATION

Is there a minimum period of time to try microdosing for before deciding either that it doesn't work, or that it just isn't right for you?

Microdosing is not for everyone. If you are microdosing to deal with a physical or mental medical condition, unless you have a strong negative reaction or experience that doesn't resolve by cutting your next dose in half, it makes sense to stay with it for at least a few weeks. Stick to the protocol you're on, keep your expectations and mindset positive, and wait and see.

WORKING WITH OTHERS

What are the advantages and disadvantages of working with others (coaches, therapists, friends, or groups) versus microdosing on your own?

Our intention in writing this book is to provide you with everything you need to know so you can safely and effectively microdose. That said, there are good reasons to work with a coach, therapist, or group of friends who support and help each other. When we work with those who know more than we do, we benefit from their knowledge and experience. And by working with others, we are more likely to stay on track.

For example, an experienced microdosing professional can help you more easily determine what for you will be the right substance, dose, and protocol. The simple fact that there is someone you can reach out to for reassurance—who will answer your questions and who you can share your success with—can make a big difference.

If you are considering working with a microdosing professional, institution, or group, here are some questions you might ask.

- What is your background and your experience?

- Do you microdose yourself? If so, what benefits have you experienced?
- What kind of experiences are common for those who are working with you?
- Can I speak with individuals who have worked with you or gone through your program?

Working with a "friend group"* can provide a nice balance between personal microdosing and working with a coach or therapist as you will be able to access the collective knowledge and wisdom of the group. Moreover, the importance of positive social reinforcement—both in maintaining a positive mindset and in keeping you to your protocol— should not be underestimated. Some friend groups sync their microdosing protocol and schedules so members can compare notes and cheer each other on. In addition, we know that being part of a social group has positive impacts on mental and physical health.[31] As more and more professionals offer services, more institutions offer support and training, and more local support groups become available, it may be to your advantage to consider these alternatives to working on your own.

Preliminaries: Introduction to Health Conditions and Symptoms Benefited

Sources of Information

Where does this information come from?

We take an interest in a condition once it's been reported by one or more individuals or has emerged in a clinical study. We then carefully read and follow up with any new information.

---

*Cultivating "friend groups" for micro- and macrodosing has been championed by Patrick Ironwood, whose Psychedelic Universe presence on the app Clubhouse has been very helpful in refining some of our ideas.

We err in favor of including remarkable results, even from a single person. As we get more examples, we review our prior findings.

For example, the initial report about the effectiveness of microdosing for the symptoms of shingles—especially for acute pain—came from an email sent to Jim from a reader in Namibia. Two more reports from individuals in Europe confirmed some of what we had understood, but not all. Several years later, Jim observed someone recovering from severe pain and diminished vitality; he learned that while the recovery *alleviated her pain and restored additional capacities,* it did not heal the root cause of her condition. More information on this case is presented later on in chapter 5's discussion of shingles on page 224.

We present as much information as we have from whatever sources we can find, without imagining that we understand the full extent or ramifications of any particular microdosing intervention.*

In every case—and we probably repeat this too often—*the correct dose for the desired improvement varies with each condition, each protocol, and most importantly, each individual.*

While individuals should make use of all the information available, they should also accept this information as *only a first approximation* of what may be right for themselves or someone they know or care for.

We present as many possibilities as seem applicable. Note: we also have included health conditions caused by negative effects of medications and treatments. Some of these are widely acknowledged, such as the emotional flatness often associated with SSRIs, while others are less often noticed and not as fully described.

We have included research whenever we can. However, research findings that focus on the statistical analysis of groups often obscure individual data, especially the more extreme individual results. Medians, means, modes, and ranges all, of course, have value. But individual cases often contain much more specific and useful information. In an obser-

---

*Or when pursuing any enhancement of abilities, wellness, or flow.

vational citizen science–informed approach, even one story helps map the currents of the ever-evolving stream of microdosing information.

Extrapolating from Single Cases

Isn't reporting improvements in medical conditions with only a case or two jumping the gun or cherry-picking?

While this question feels somewhat accusatory, we try to limit our reporting to observations and not generalize beyond them. In that practice, we closely follow the lines of modern science.

Throughout this book we stress the value, even the necessity, of self-reports. What is not well-known is that first-person accounts have been considered a fundamental and essential methodology—especially for understanding inner states—for centuries. The editorial boards of medical journals regularly approve articles discussing and describing single cases, especially in areas of new disease discoveries and treatments.

At least since the founding of the Royal Society of London in 1660, lengthy reporting—including self-reporting—of individual cases has been one of the primary methods used in medical and other observational sciences. The Royal Society's motto is *Nullius in verba,* meaning "Nothing on authority." It is "an expression of the determination of Fellows to withstand the domination of authority and to verify all statements by an appeal to facts determined by experiment."[32] The readers of the Society's published proceedings were invited to repeat the experiments themselves and to write in such evidence that confirmed or denied them.[33]

Extensive examination of individual cases, followed by group observations of the same condition or enhancement, is precisely what led to current best practices and our collective knowledge pool.

As microdosing has become more widely used, social media has become a useful method for helping to evaluate single cases. The Reddit microdosing subreddit, for example, has about 275,000 members who quickly consider, evaluate, challenge, and request supporting information about new uses. Other archives of general psychedelic experiences include the massive files of Erowid—which roughly translates to "Earth Wisdom"—a repository of tens of thousands of explorations of all kinds.

Working with Minors

A few of the health conditions described affect mainly children and minors. What's the best way to work with questions of legality, ethics, and consent?

The default way to deal with legality, ethics, and consent is to not give any medications to minors,* and, perhaps by extension, elderly people and others who cannot give informed consent.

While that's the conventional answer and the "easy way out," it flies in the face of the truth: parents will do most anything to help their children, no matter the obstacles in their way. As researchers and explorers, our advice when asked—and we have been asked often over the years—has been this: "We can't recommend what you should decide to do. As human beings talking to other human beings, we will give you all the information we can to assist you in making the most informed decision you possibly can."

This book is neither a textbook nor a rulebook. It is more like a travel guide to the country of microdosing. It's a descriptive guide to what you may find there, based on what others who have already traveled there have found.

When we do have specific information related to minors, it is mentioned in the discussion of that particular condition (see, for example, our reports on ADHD and autism on pages 109 and 166).

---

*Children's brains are not fully developed, which is why so many medications are not recommended for them. However, we know of children raised in South American ayahuasca churches who are given small amounts of ayahuasca from a very early age. When tested against contemporaries in their same village, they do better in school, have fewer physical problems, and are generally healthier than their non-ayahuasca-taking companions. We have some additional observations on the effect of microdosing on mothers and their children in chapter 4's discussion of women's health.

Continuing Medications

Can I continue medications that work well for me while I'm microdosing?

Based on individual microdosing reports and other sources, we have included an appendix (page 299) of hundreds of substances—medications, supplements, herbs, and more—reported to be safe for use while microdosing. (Also a few substances that are contraindicated.) This is useful information for the increasing number of people who take multiple medications and also wish to explore microdosing.

[3]

Enhanced Abilities, Wellness, and Flow

When I microdose, I feel better. Colors are brighter.
I am happier and more pleasant to be around.
I think I'm funnier and more creative.
—Paul Stamets (2025)

Why discuss "Enhanced Abilities, Wellness, and Flow" before turning to mental and physical conditions?

We are as excited and focused on the possibilities of microdosing for improved parenting or martial arts as we are with benefits for depression or pain control. This chapter on "Enhanced Abilities, Wellness, and Flow" covers general interests that apply to everyone, including creative endeavors, work-related skills and capacities, physical passions and pursuits, inner work and relaxation, time spent in relationships, and so on. As "The Viability of Microdosing Psychedelics as a Strategy to Enhance Cognition and Well-Being: An Early Review" puts it, and as our findings and reports reinforce, "Exploratory evidence published to date indicates a variety of benefits reported by microdosers including improvements in mood, focus, and creativity" (Bornemann, 2020).

The psychedelic mindset currently derived from research and clinical reports and agreed upon by the scientific and financial communities— and coming almost entirely from the results of high-dose studies—is focused mainly on depression, trauma-related conditions, and mental illness. The psychedelic renaissance or revival has not yet focused on *healthy uses* or on *spiritual awakening,* both of which were also part of the psychedelic era of the 1960s. Instead, medical use has taken the spotlight in the center ring of psychedelic focus. But now two smaller rings on either side—healthy uses and spiritual awakening—are gradually becoming visible and receiving favorable notice.[1] We are starting with these positive uses to help cultivate a broad and open-minded context for the consideration of mental and physical conditions in the following two chapters.

Cognitive Enhancement

Does the idea of "fine tuning," as you'd do with a car, apply here?

That's a good metaphor, very close to what actually occurs.

One way to describe microdosing's overall effects is that it improves the body's various operating systems. It is equally as useful for improved creativity, performance, or interpersonal relations as it is for those seeking better mental and physical health, including reducing pain and suffering of all kinds.

In 2015, *Rolling Stone* published "How LSD Microdosing Became the Hot New Business Trip,"[2] an article about a young Silicon Valley design engineer that was widely quoted and commented on, both in print and online. Some of the stories were about microdosing becoming a new fad in Silicon Valley. To this day, the notion that microdosing is most popular among Bay Area tech workers remains a staple of microdosing lore.

Within a few years, it became a self-fulfilling prophecy. Reporters looking for new stories about successful startups and fast-growing larger companies would often report that more and more people were microdosing to stay competitive. In a video interview, Tim Ferriss really did say, "The billionaires I know, almost without exception, use hallucinogens on a regular basis."[3] More people explored psychedelics and more found that microdosing worked for them.

The "tune-up" metaphor is a good one, then, because when you tune up a car's engine, you're not replacing one part with a new one so much as you are ensuring that each part is working at peak efficiency and in concert with all the others.

Reports from healthy people who consistently microdose talk about improved mood, energy, and productivity, a heightened appreciation of nature, often a shift toward healthier eating and better sleep, and even improved sexual relations. In the long run, these ways of improving overall health and functioning may become the dominant reason that most people work with microdosing. As for cognitive enhancement in particular, see later entries in this section on creativity enhanced, focus improved, math and coding, and writing and playing music.

Creativity Enhanced (Art)

Many artists and musicians talk about taking acid. Is it their art that's better, or just their opinion of it?

Early on, an artist wrote Jim and Sophia Korb to let them know (in somewhat unkind terms) that he had tried a microdose, but to him it seemed worthless—he felt no effects, and no benefits. Writing him back, Sophia mentioned that microdosing initially disappointed some people with considerable psychedelic experience because they mistakenly imagined it would be like a small version of their high-dose experiences.

His response was not exactly an apology but, upon reflection, he acknowledged that on the microdosing day he'd completed two paintings he'd had difficulty with for weeks, and he'd been able to work "full out" for longer than he had in months.

Many artists who have creatively engaged, either on high doses or very soon thereafter, have felt their psychedelic experiences led to major improvements in their art. From our point of view, and from the point of view of art critics, after someone substantially changes their style, color palette, or subject matter, it's very hard to say if what results is an improvement.

Microdosing has about the same effect on artists as it does on writers, coders, and mathematicians. This includes making it generally easier to render what exists in one's mind onto paper, canvas, ceramic, or computer screen. Microdosing may not improve or change the final product or quality but it increases the ease and subjective pleasure of creation.

Creativity Enhanced (Writing)

On several podcasts, I've heard Jim say that "microdosing is great for first drafts." Any evidence?

Not only has Jim spoken about it on podcasts but he suggested it directly to several journalists interviewing him. In what might be called instant research, a few took the suggestion seriously and later said they did find they were writing more easily and were better able to come up with what they needed in much less time than usual. One or two college journalists wrote about their first experience in their articles.

When anxiety is lowered, intellectual flexibility increases, and when emotional concerns become less intrusive, staying focused on writing becomes easier. People don't report that the writing itself is necessarily better, but they do say that they can move into producing better first drafts with less effort.

Focus

What are people talking about when they say that microdosing gives them more focus?

Focus doesn't have a quantity, like salt. So people who talk about having more focus probably mean they had better focus, or could stay focused longer.

Two key qualities are involved with focus: an increased ability not to be distracted from a task or activity, as well as the total amount of time that one can spend fully focused.

Flow, a concept popularized by Mihaly Csikszentmihalyi, is the term often used for being in the most focused and creative state of mind. Microdosers commonly report that they can focus more easily, and, once engaged, stay in flow longer.

Takeaway: With microdosing, people are less distractible, have better concentration, and are able to stay longer with any given task.

> I had more energy and did a lot more, but
> what was wonderful was that despite my
> usual habit of looking at a task and saying,
> "I'll do it later," another part of me pushed that
> thought aside and I just did the thing
> right then and there.
> —Heard at a social gathering, from someone
> just beginning to microdose

Food Choices

Can microdosing help me make better food choices?

Given how many millions of dollars are spent so you'd rather purchase a bag of potato chips for a few dollars than spend far less money to cut up and fry some potatoes, the reports we received on this were initially surprising. While very few people initially looked to microdosing to improve their food habits, we found that many of those who reported to us were unaware—until they reviewed the results of a month of microdosing—that they were eating healthier foods. This was not their intention, and not even on their lists of possible outcomes. Regardless, it seemed the natural wisdom of their bodies now had more votes about what to eat than before.

Early on, Jim received daily reports from an individual who decided to use microdosing while undertaking extensive personal journaling to help him overcome his primary concerns: compulsive gambling and excessive pot smoking. He also had a junk-food diet.

At one point, however, as he somewhat incredulously reported, "I was out with the kids and my girlfriend, and we went to a restaurant. I looked at the menu, and, by God, I actually *wanted* a salad."

If one of your intentions is to make better food choices, it's likely that microdosing will facilitate it. And even if it isn't one of your intentions, you just might find that without any particular hoopla or effort, you are indeed making better, wiser, and more sensible food choices.

Grades and Academics

If I get better grades while I'm microdosing, and then I stop, will I still stay smarter?

From what we now know, an honest and accurate answer is a definite "maybe."

We have many reports from people at various levels in academia—from high school to postdoctoral programs—stating that microdosing improved their focus and memory, lowered test anxiety, and helped overcome procrastination in writing papers and preparing presentations. We have very few reports as to whether such improvements—once microdosing was stopped—persisted or declined.

We also have a good number of reports on people who microdosed at one point in their lives and achieved their intentions, then stopped. At a later time, for different reasons, they chose to microdose again.

For example, one early adopter with considerable learning difficulties began microdosing in her senior year of high school. She upped her grade average, got accepted by the college she wanted to attend, and was offered a good scholarship. In college, she found herself struggling again. She returned to microdosing and ended up an honors student. She is currently completing an advanced degree in counseling.

We have clear evidence that people with ADHD have been able to improve some of the skills they needed in school over and above what they'd achieved with medication alone. If as you're microdosing you develop better study habits, learn to take better class notes, or perhaps improve your computer skills, you will retain more of your gains than someone who only takes advantage of the effects of microdoses in the moment and doesn't lock in any new skills or study habit improvements.

Short answer: There likely is some decline in mental capacity once microdosing is stopped, but if, while microdosing, you consciously improve your skills, then more will be retained.

Happy (Truly)

Does microdosing make people genuinely happy, and if so, does it last even when people stop?

Early on, Jim and his then-collaborator Sophia Korb created MicrodosingPsychedelics.com to answer the most commonly asked questions about substances, doses, protocols, limitations, and so on. In exchange for the information they were given, website visitors were asked (if they decided to microdose) to fill out a very short daily checklist about positive and negative emotions, and to add any notes they thought were of interest. They were requested to reflect on their experience after thirty days and send in a report. Eventually, there were more than 1,500 responses from fifty-one countries. Of the first seven hundred reports analyzed, at least half were from people with treatment-resistant depression.

The checklist* included twenty emotions, ten of which were posi-

---

*The widely adopted PANAS (Positive and Negative Affect Schedule) was used; it will be discussed later under depression in chapter 4.

tive, such as "cheerful" and "enthusiastic," and ten that were negative, like "sad" or "depressed."

There are many published studies showing that when antidepressants are effective, they take the sting out of negative events, and people are better able to cope as actual and psychologically generated sorrows are more easily tolerated. The shadow side of removing the sting is that, for many people, antidepressants mute positive feelings.

After microdosing, about 80 percent of the depressed group reported that they were less depressed overall, many of them significantly so. Their negative emotions were far less disturbing—very much like favorable responses to antidepressants. However, their positive emotions increased to the same extent or greater than their negative emotions had declined.

With SSRIs people are less sad, but in many cases they are also less glad. Those who microdosed were also less sad, *and* they were significantly more glad. They reported they felt much more like the selves they knew before they became depressed.

An old friend and former student of Jim's wrote: "For the first time in thirty-one years, I am off all antidepressants. Also, for the first time in ever so long, I have my full span of emotions. I'm embarrassing people because I now cry so easily, but often it's because I'm so happy that I can't contain it."

In short, people microdosing for depression—some very early in their microdosing experience—feel as if they have returned to a normal self, and a happier one.

Now let's consider whether these feelings of normality and happiness are maintained without continual microdosing support.

As is true of many questions about how long various changes last, sustaining ongoing happiness without further microdosing is not well explored. A woman artist wrote Jim to celebrate her own recovery from long-term depression. A few months later, she wrote again. She had recommended microdosing to a number of her friends who also suffered from long-term depression. She related that some of them, after microdosing for several months, had stopped and felt no return of their depression. Another group also were not depressed, but after stopping for several weeks, their depression began to return. Returning to microdosing, they found relief.

The woman wanted to know why there was a difference between these two groups. Jim asked her if there were any differences that she had observed. After puzzling over things for a while, she noted that her friends who stopped and maintained their happiness had lives that were working, while most of her friends who chose to resume were in difficult or stressful life situations.

Draw your own conclusions.

Language Learning

As a kid I learned two foreign languages—it was easy for me. But not now. Would microdosing potentially help me get back that capacity?

If language learning is simply seen as another type of learning, it's not surprising that microdosing could make it easier or more efficient. We know that microdosing enhances neuroplasticity, which among other things means enhancing the brain's capacity to encode new learning.

Quite a few of our real-world reports suggest it *does* make a big difference. For example, "I am English, married to a Norwegian, and we live in a small town in Norway. Learning Norwegian has been difficult, but has become much easier since I've started microdosing."

A post by Chris Eubanks in Medium.com showcases an interesting method. In "My Experience Microdosing to Learn a Language,"[4] Chris watches the same YouTube video thirty to fifty times in a row before reaching 75 percent understanding and moving on to the next video.

"I decided to take 1/8 of my normal 'full trip' LSD dose to see what would happen. . . . Everything felt smoother. I watched the same Finnish videos over and over again and kept a tally sheet. Normally, I study Finnish 3 hours per day, but on my first day microdosing, I studied for 12 hours. . . . While microdosing, I am much more engaged with the language, so I can put longer hours into studying it."

Or consider this report from a Reddit user:

"I generally struggle with maintaining focus and my attention tends to wander quite quickly. Although even without md, studying coding has been much easier for me to focus on than most of my past endeavors.

No md: I'm working on understanding a particular part of a language and its function, then, as my learning grows, I'll start to see how it slots into the bigger picture.

With md: What I'm learning seems to fit into the bigger picture almost seamlessly, so I'm understanding *why* things are working much faster.

Side note: I take my md in the mornings and do struggle to get my thoughts focused for the first few hours. The latter half of day 1 and entire day 2, I really like for the reasons mentioned above."[5]

Which psychedelic works best? If you look through Reddit, LSD is slightly favored. A typical comment states:

"From my personal experience, mushroom microdosing gives you a lot of energy and focus. LSD microdosing does the same, except you pick up new things more quickly. You just need to experiment for yourself, it's different for everyone. See what works for you."[6]

In sum, if microdosing helps with learning in general, language learning would be included. Pourquoi pas prendre une chance? ¿Por qué no arriesgarse?

Longevity

Can microdosing help me live longer?

The momentum of the psychedelic revival has sparked interest in those dedicated to extending and maximizing human lifespan. A 2023 article in *The Guardian*, "'Long-Lost Best Friends': The Longevity Movement Finds Psychedelics," describes the "crossover" between these two worlds:

> Longevity proponents . . . offered a few explanations—most simply, that psychedelics could improve health or lifespan by alleviating the symptoms of mental illness. There are some early suggestions that psychedelics can have physical effects like reducing inflammation or increasing brain chemicals and connections, which might affect longevity too. If psychedelics help mental health, and mental health is part of both health and lifespan extension, then psychedelics might be an important longevity tool.[7]

In "The Curious Connection Between Psychedelics and Longevity," Zach Haigney makes the comparison that "psychedelics are to the mind what longevity drugs are to the body."[8] He concludes:

> The drugs we may eventually see come out of longevity science will be accelerants of DRM [defense, repair, and maintenance] processes in the same way that psychedelics are accelerants of neuroplastic changes. In this way, longevity drugs are to the immune system what psychedelics are to the brain.[9]

Math and Coding

My college math grades are low. Could microdosing help?

There's no magic here. You still need to do all the work. However, microdosing might help you do what a lot of others have done. We have reports from high school, college, and graduate students saying that microdosing raised their grades. One Dartmouth math major wrote, "I was getting by and struggling. Microdosing lowered my anxiety and helped me focus. I decided to take the hardest course in the catalog. I sailed through it without anxiety. A couple of my math-major friends are now also microdosing."

Here is a similar statement on r/microdosing[10] by someone familiar with microdosing:

> "I'm a PhD student, not a stoner. I've microdosed LSD and
> psilocybin. They are wonderful tools for a mathematician.
> They provide you with a very clean energy and open up your
> mind to new thoughts. I've had many new ideas come to me
> due to psychedelics."

Another Reddit user, who had just discovered microdosing, posted:

> "For the past week, microdosing [psilocybin] shrooms at
> just below threshold (0.2–0.5 g). I can easily understand
> the 'big picture' when working with a particular API
> [application program interface] or when making major
> structural/refactoring changes to one. . . . Cause and effect
> between concepts are understood incredibly quickly. . . . My
> thinking process is more 'uniform' when thinking about a
> concept or working on a thought."[11]

Finally, a young man at a San Francisco Psychedelic Society meetup, responding to a question asked by a member, said: "I only microdose when I have a coding problem."

Music (Creating and Performing)

I'm a professional musician and I know and appreciate how smoking pot changes my playing. Will microdosing affect me differently?

Back when the effects of microdosing were first being discovered, a letter (not an email) came in: "I'm not a professional musician, but a group of us get together to sing and play. I can't tell if my playing is improved, though it might be, but what is real obvious is that when I've microdosed, I remember more songs and many more verses of songs I thought I'd forgotten."

In other reports, people often say that their performance anxiety is much less or no longer a problem. The changes reported include overall capacity, emotional stability, and physical facility rather than musicianship per se.

Short answer: You will likely play better, and even more likely, you will enjoy playing more.

Sexual Enhancement

How about microdosing in bed?

> After microdosing about 4 weeks I have become
> consistently horny, sex drive like a 19-year-old.
> Anyone else experience this? Is it temporary?
> How do I maintain it? lol
> —On Reddit, around Valentine's Day 2024

A brief email report early on was our first clue: "If it gets out what this does for your libido, you'll have a real product."

We have seen quite a few reports from people whose sex life has improved while microdosing. This may be because many people find microdosing inherently energizing.

Sex in human beings is a combination of physiology and psychology. What we know is that microdosing improves sexual relations between partners. What we don't know is to what degree such improvement can be attributed to being more caring—with better communication and more spontaneous cuddling—versus improved blood flow capacity and sensitivity for arousal. Sexuality is a good example where you can't simply extrapolate from laboratory animals or laboratory research to human beings.

It may not be so much a question of microdosing changing or increasing your libido or sex drive or facilitating lasting longer or having more intense orgasms. It may be that it simply makes you more sensitive and aware of your partner's needs. Some people have reported either their whole system being more sensitive, so sex was more pleasurable, or finding that their relationship was more pleasurable, so that it became easier both to give and receive pleasure. That is, it's not that there is more testosterone but there does seem to be more oxytocin and therefore more connectedness.

Also, we know from life itself that people who feel better about themselves—physically healthier and more emotionally content—are better listeners and better in bed. It may also be that increased libido actually is, at least in part, what's driving better sex.

Sleep Quality

Can microdosing improve my sleep and sleep quality?

Generally healthy people who reported improved overall functioning (greater mental clarity and emotional equilibrium, improved relationships, and improved physical functioning) often mention better or longer sleep. Until recently, however, we had no data beyond that.

In 2023, a double-blind placebo-controlled microdosing study of eighty healthy men taking either ten micrograms of LSD or a placebo, monitored over forty-nine days, showed significant sleep differences between the microdose group and the placebo group.[12] Each participant wore a sleep monitor that measured not only total sleep time but the amount of sleep in each stage. On the Fadiman protocol, the microdosing group slept approximately twenty-four minutes longer, not on the night of the actual dose but one night later. The researchers' analysis showed that the microdosing group went to bed earlier, then awakened at the same time as the placebo group. Moreover, a considerable amount of the extra sleep was in maximally restorative deep sleep.

The researchers speculated on the benefits of this added sleep, suggesting, for example, that it might be part of the reason that other microdosing studies show improved depression scores. For our purposes, it is enough to note that, in this sample, microdosing taken in the morning led to more sleep on the second night.

Social Microdoses

My new girlfriend invited me to a party. When I said I'd pick up a six-pack, she said it was "mushrooms only." What's going on?

While we won't cover "social microdosing" in any detail, we note that microdoses are being served at parties, after-work get-togethers, friend gatherings, celebrations, and even weddings. Microdoses are becoming a viable alternative for a generation turning away from alcohol. Instead of alcohol, the psilocybin-infused chocolates offered to guests encourage them to enjoy the event and one another.

Prior to this trend, as cannabis has become more accepted in state after state, alcohol sales have diminished. We leave it to others to discuss the correlation of the increasing availability of cannabis and the decline of drinking, but we are struck by how quickly microdosing is establishing itself as another viable alternative.

In a recent article in *Refinery29*, Fortesa Latifi reports that while people still talk mainly about the mental health benefits of microdosing, they also "microdose for a much simpler reason: fun." Her article continues:

> Shrooms appear to fit into the lives of those who want to cut back on the booze, but still socialize and let loose. "A microdose is a nice balance where you're still getting a buzz," Helena, 31 . . . says. "But when it's over you don't have a hangover or feel groggy." . . . Bennett, 31 . . . says . . . "You don't have to deal with hangovers or making stupid or embarrassing decisions while you're drunk." . . . Helena [continues], "A lot of my friends have gotten into it. . . . It used to feel very taboo, but now it's becoming a thing." Bennett says, "If it's enjoyed responsibly, I feel like the harm is way less."[13]

Additionally, microdoses are consciously being used to minimize drinking at weddings. All too many of us have memories of a beautiful ceremony or party being ruined by a friend of the groom or bride who tells embarrassing stories before losing their balance and pancaking onto the floor. So, instead of serving champagne, some serve microdoses in chocolates. One enterprising chocolatier in Southern California reports selling five thousand pieces a month for weddings from as far back as 2021.

In Northern California, which also has its share of microdose chocolatiers, a respected herbalist puts together combinations of herbs plus psilocybin mushrooms on request. People sip on a one-ounce microdose herbal tonic or elixir, assured that they won't have any of the troubling gastric pains sometimes associated with taking psilocybin in capsules or in chocolate, plus they receive the synergistic benefits of the herbs. Reviews have been positive: "Your magical potion was just the medicine for our party. People felt elated, trippy, groovy, social, present, and connected—it was quite a change from a party focused on alcohol as the intoxicant."[14]

Uses have expanded well beyond parties: "The moms of Marin all love the potion! It seems to be the cure for the stresses of parenting and makes our time with our children more enjoyable and present. Personally, I've also been sleeping better, even on the days that I don't take it."[15]

Sports and Athletics

In 1970, Dock Ellis pitched a no-hitter for the Pittsburgh Pirates very high on a lot of LSD. Can regular people use microdoses to play better?

Success in sports—from weight lifting and skydiving to baseball and marathon running—comes from a mixture of speed, strength, coordination, endurance, strategy, and cooperation, as well as heightened sensory acuity or "enhanced awareness." As the first six of these factors are self-explanatory, let's begin with an extended example of enhanced awareness.

Saying someone has "eyes in the back of their head"—an ability called "scopaesthesia"—is a metaphor for enhanced awareness. While there is no scientific agreement about this capacity, its existence is common knowledge throughout professional sports. Microdosing apparently makes it easier to notice and act in concert with the intention of others. A martial arts report from a jujitsu practitioner on Reddit provides a detailed description:

> "I'm a Brazilian Jiu-Jitsu practitioner, and I've been training
> for about 5 years before I actually started using mushrooms
> for enhancement. . . . I've only been using mushrooms for
> about 1 month, and I've had a noticeable difference in a few

areas. I microdose 3 to 4 times a week and take at least three consecutive days off.

One of the biggest areas I've had a noticeable improvement in is my speed of decision making and reaction time. Brazilian jiu-jitsu is one of those sports where every decision you make can lead to a different outcome. Knowing when to make the decision, knowing when to pull the trigger, and when to hold back, is a big part of the game. I found that while microdosing, the time period in between thinking of a move and actually performing the move and or executing a counter is almost eliminated. My body just performs the action as I think it.

Another big difference is that I get into a flow state much faster. . . . I find that with the mushrooms . . . my mind just completely clears itself and focuses solely on one objective.

The third area that I noticed a huge change in would be my actual creativity when it comes to applying moves. I tend to take much higher risks without thinking much about the consequences . . . allowing my body to experience what it's like to move uninterrupted by my thoughts."[16]

The importance of enhanced awareness, in combination with the other better-understood factors noted above—speed, strength, endurance, coordination, strategy, and cooperation—differs between various sports. A study of more than a hundred individuals who posted microdosing reports on YouTube concluded:

Athletic performance and exercising benefits of microdosing were exemplified by practitioners of many different sports and activities including ice hockey, basketball, freestyle climbing, MMA, and long-distance trail running. Increased energy, focus, coordination, prevision, and overall motivation were typical benefits attributed to the use of microdosing in sports and physical exercise.[17]

Let's look at a few specific sports where we have reports of microdosing affecting performance.

Kickboxing

Kickboxing was discussed when the popular podcaster Joe Rogan interviewed Dennis McKenna on microdosing psilocybin:

> Joe: One of the things that I'm aware of is kickboxers using microdosing. A good buddy of mine who is using it says he can see things happen before they happen—it's almost like he was reading people's minds before they are about to do something.
>
> Dennis: Even on microdosing? That's very interesting.
>
> Joe: Yes. In the intense environment of sparring and the kinetic physical action of kickboxing he is seeing what people are going to do before they do it in a way that he was never able to do "on the natch."[18]

Volleyball

A college student reported, "I'm not sure I played any better, but I could feel what the whole team was doing. And so, I could anticipate things. Basically, my strategy improved; I could do what the team needed to do much better than I had before."

Distance Running

A middle-aged man wrote that he ran faster than usual on days when he microdosed, with no more effort. Jim asked for more information. The man responded: "In two weeks, I'll be running a half marathon in a race. I'll let you know how it goes." Several weeks later, his report noted: "I'm excited to let you know that I took 20 minutes off the time from my last race 5 months ago. This was the best time I've had in the past ten years. Thank you for your work."

Microdosing apparently improves overall physical capacity. This includes the pleasure we experience when our body is doing its very best. One martial artist publicly summed up the results of his microdosing: "I used to win silver medals, now I win golds."

Vision Improvement

Do people experience better eyesight after starting to microdose?

Microdosing often improves vision during the hours when the microdose is most active, and it has been used in a number of indigenous societies to improve visual acuity for hunting. Vision also improves when high doses are taken. Jim recalls:

> When I was learning to be a psychedelic guide in the 1960s, we were aware that during a high-dose session people had better vision. They had an enhanced capacity to see detail, near or far. One of the best indicators we had that a person was returning to normal consciousness in the late afternoon of a session day was when they reached for their glasses.

We did not, however, anticipate that any improved vision would be retained. The following reports about both brief and long-term improvements open a new area for research.

- "I grabbed my phone to turn off the sound settings while I was trying to relax into the experience. Without thinking, I shoved my eyeglasses up on my nose because I normally can see only a dark knob in my hand without them. The surprise was that it was not only not a dark knob, it was hazy and distorted *until*

I took my glasses off, then everything was clear as day. . . . The effect started waning as the experience wore off."

- "I remember having a conversation with my eyes and my brain . . . like, really brain? You have the capability of allowing me to see clearly without glasses, but you choose not to? Thanks guy."
- "My eyesight had gotten worse in the past half a decade, but when I'm microdosing . . . I definitely have sharper visual acuity! . . . I see much brighter, notice increased textural detail, and can focus on distance a bit better."

The above reports show vision effects while microdosing. The following ones suggest that microdosing can not only improve visual acuity but for some people, the improvement lingers and in some cases stabilizes.

- "I noticed for about a week after a 0.3 gram mushroom dose, I didn't need my glasses to read."
- "I had my visual acuity assessed at the optometrist after microdosing. I did better than I usually do."
- "My eyesight has improved on my prescription."
- "Vision has been 20/40 for years. Went to my optometrist to see if I needed new glasses. He tested me, and I was seeing 20/30. Got a prescription for new glasses but then remembered I'd microdosed that morning. Canceled new glasses, booked another appointment, and he tested me again two weeks later (nonmicrodosing day). Told me the new prescription was not right. But then—surprise to both of us—my eyes were even better than 20/30. Looks like my vision has stabilized and is better. Wow!"

These reports raise questions as to what actually changes in the visual system during microdosing, and how to explain why, for some people, improved vision is retained. No answers yet.

Work Quality Improvement

People in Silicon Valley and other tech centers apparently use micro-dosing for better focus and creativity. What's the downside?

Whether it's exploitative or not, many workplace amenities are *not* there out of employers' generosity or goodness of heart but as ways to improve overall results and achieve a better bottom line. These "things" include air-conditioning, comfortable chairs, coffee breaks, a lunch period long enough to do more than eat, and so on. At the peak of Silicon Valley's dot-com boom in 1999–2000, companies vied with one another to make work as pleasant as possible, with gourmet meals, on-site child care, laundry, dry-cleaning services, and more.

When it's suggested to those who microdose at work that they're being exploited, they rarely agree. Instead, they point out that being productive with less anxiety and more creativity is a pleasure in and of itself. In addition, there are many reports from people in dead-end, uncomfortable, underpaid, or pointless jobs. They generally report that while their situation is the same as it was prior to microdosing, they are (a) less unhappy and more tolerant, (b) no less interested in improving their lives and no less aware of injustice, economic or otherwise, and (c) in a better internal position to deal with whatever comes next.

Being better at work, or being better able to cope when at work, are common responses across occupations, industries, and even countries. And yes, some people also find it easier to quit if necessary. They feel more confident in their ability to find a more suitable job, and less worried and anxious in the meantime.

[4]

Current Findings
of Special Interest

This chapter presents findings in six areas where microdosing can possibly make a major impact. The first five sections review the evidence for microdosing aiding healing and recovery, while the last looks at enhancing the health of women during pregnancy, breastfeeding, and early parenting. The six sections are:

- **ADHD**: The number of cases has almost doubled in the last few years, with lifelong medication being suggested for children as young as three.
- **Depression:** The most reported mental illness worldwide. Not only was it exacerbated by the pandemic, but the most widely used medications are not terribly good.
- **Long COVID:** There are millions of cases in the US alone, but generally few effective treatments.
- **Pain Management:** Studies as well as reports from users confirm the value of microdosing for pain control and feeling better generally.

- **Tapering Off Medications:** It is difficult and sometimes dangerous to stop the use of many medications. Microdosing apparently makes it easier and safer.
- **Women's Health:** During pregnancy and early childbirth, the typical medical advice is to stop taking many medications. There are no recommendations as to taking microdoses, but a first survey* suggests microdosing to be health enhancing.

We have more information about these six areas—a wide range of reports, and early research findings—than on most others. For each, we see microdosing as a clear alternative to what is currently widely available.

ADHD
(Attention Deficit/Hyperactivity Disorder)

Adderall Alternative

Adderall controls my ADHD symptoms, but I hate the side effects and may be addicted. Is microdosing an alternative? (I'm twenty-seven.)

To answer this seemingly simple question, we need to understand the nature of ADHD. Doing so brings up a number of issues, including:

- The almost universal use of central nervous system stimulants as prescribed treatments
- A massive uptick in ADHD prescriptions (more so for women) over the last few years
- The positive and negative effects of current medications
- The reality that ADHD drugs are a multibillion-dollar industry

---

*The results reported on women's health reflect the first major survey of microdosing focused solely on pregnancy, breastfeeding, and early parenting, an area curiously neglected from the sixties until now.

Before we approach these issues, let's review a spectrum of reports from those choosing to microdose to address ADHD. Most of the reports were from individuals on prescribed medications, but, to start, we have several reports from those coping on their own.

Reports

ADHD Symptoms—No Medications

- "Not diagnosed, but have had issues/symptoms characteristic of ADD/ADHD. I don't believe my big house remodeling project would be going this well if not for the help of microdosing. It could be circumstantial, but even with nine workers coming at me with questions, decisions needed, and a flood of activity, I'm making good choices and managing even my regular job deadlines while also feeling confident. This has not been me for a long time."

- "I haven't been diagnosed with ADHD, but have had lots of symptoms that have almost completely gone away now. My focus is so much better at work. I used to have days I would get tons done, then the next day no focus at all. This isn't an issue any more—I can bring my focus to what needs doing despite my mood. I am (dare I say) not avoidant of challenges in the same way. I can put my anxiety aside and crack on. My thoughts are less scattered. I am able to keep my house in order without any issue, I am not as messy as I was. I see things that need doing and do them without the overwhelm."

- "I used to have a dining room table covered in stuff and it overwhelmed me where to put it all! I found it so hard to be tidy or figure out where to put stuff—and there was always *more* stuff, especially the kids' stuff. Now I don't really think about it, and I just clear it up! My memory is better. I can handle a calendar better and forget things less. The multitude of thoughts that overwhelmed me are less intrusive. Greater clarity. Wow! Makes me realize as I write this that things have shifted a lot in my functioning—it's all been slow and incremental improvements with no intentional effort on my part, a natural outcome of the microdosing."

ADHD Improved with Microdosing

- "I have found microdosing mushrooms to be the most beneficial tool yet in dealing with my ADHD. At 38, life with ADHD has been very challenging for me. The thoughts never stop, and they're quite often self-defeating, antagonistic and painful. Some days it would feel like my mind was on fire. Then I tried microdosing. The noise stopped. Altogether stopped. Actual silence, observable silence."
- "MD [microdosing] to me is comparable to the positive parts of Adderall without all of the horrible downsides. I know some people are fine on Adderall, but for me it made me severely depressed, took away my personality, couldn't have sex, etc. On an LSD MD I get the improved focus or interest without any of the other side effects."
- "It is a little harder for me to focus on days off [not dosing] and I sometimes think 'this would be easier/more enjoyable if I did MD,' but I'm still able to work and get things done. If anything, MD allowed me to recognize my thought patterns that lead to procrastination, and I am aware of that on days off."
- "LSD is like the perfect all day lasting stimulant I always needed but was never prescribed."
- "For me it replaces two medications, Adderall, and the nerve pain medication I used to take, Neurontin."
- "I used LSD to get off a decade-plus Adderall prescription."

ADHD Improved but with Clear Limitations

- "It's done wonders for my depression, anxiety, and to a lesser extent OCD, but my good old ADHD is still going nuts. If anything, the relief from anxiety has made it worse. That's a tradeoff I'd make any day though."
- "I don't even really MD anymore after doing it for years. It seems like my depression and anxiety are gone. All I'm left with is the ADHD symptoms, which I had before."

Blending Microdosing with Prescription Medications

- "I found microdosing LSD only by itself doesn't help. But Vyvanse with microdosing has been helping me out. MD'ing helps with depression and makes me calmer. Vyvanse helps my focus."
- "My ADHD is pretty severe, so I still take Adderall, but microdosing with LSD definitely helps. It completely eliminates the side effects I get from Adderall and reduces the amount I need, plus I get all the other benefits of microdosing like increased focus, motivation, better mood, and being more social and less anxious."
- "Can confirm on efficacy. I still take Adderall though. I did decrease my usage, so I'm basically down to 1/3 the dose of what I'm prescribed."
- "Just starting with shrooms/truffles. I've been trying it for almost 2 weeks, but I sometimes take methylphenidate [Ritalin] with it as it is not completely working for my ADHD. But I love this stuff, and will keep taking it. It makes me more relaxed; it makes me so aware of my feelings and thoughts of myself and others (growth on a deep level). I also feel less of a comedown from the medication."

- "It doesn't help the ADHD symptoms themselves, but definitely helps me accept my brain for what it is, and I rely much less on my Vyvanse because of that."
- "On days when I MD I don't need anything else. And the days that I forget my ADD stack [of medications], I honestly don't miss them."

Specific Changes

- "As far as sex drive, it's not so much an issue of lack of drive with Adderall, but a lack of ability. Lol! On MD I just feel normal drive and ability to pull through."
- "Most noticeable effect for me has been in my creativity. I do a lot of spiritual writing. I seem to be able to tap into and create more easily and readily. It's also increased my problem solving. I'm more open from a social aspect as well. Being able to connect much easier with other people without having to actively try."
- "I started MD for severe depression. I went the pharma route when I was a teenager (now 43), and it had no long-term positive effects. Basically, a MD of 0.2 grams dried mushrooms every 3 days for six months reduced my depression to occasional sadness. A 'side effect' of the MDing is that my focus and attention span has increased 100-fold."

Dosing in the Evening

- "Lately I've been taking it after work so the evenings are more peaceful, and I sleep better at night, making the next day better."
- "MD makes my evening better giving me more confidence, improving my overall mental health [and] preparing me for the next day, and next days are usually better, making me think more positively and deal with the world where I don't fit in."

When Effects Are Felt

- "The energetic effect is within the hour of taking it for me. And it's not stimulant type energy, it's more subtle and I don't really notice it until I realize I am much less hesitant to start on something and have increased focus."

Research Reports

With research studies confirming individual reports, microdosing becomes a realistic alternative—or perhaps an adjunct—to other ADHD treatments.

For example, a study of two hundred individuals diagnosed with ADHD tested the efficacy of a monthlong microdosing regimen.[1] Half the sample were taking prescription ADHD medications, while the other half were not. After one month, almost all individuals in both groups showed significant improvement in their ADHD symptoms. Almost all individuals in both groups showed approximately the same level of improvement. Although the group on medications showed less improvement for the first two weeks, they caught up by month's end.

Another study comparing microdosing with conventional treatments found "microdosing was rated more effective than conventional therapy for diagnoses of ADHD/ADD."[2] And in a third study, of 233 adults with ADHD or ADHD-like symptoms who already intended to start microdosing, data was collected two weeks and four weeks after they started. "[We] found positive changes in mindfulness, specifically the mindfulness facets description and non-judging of inner experience, and in the personality trait neuroticism."[3]

ADHD: Additional Considerations

The following material is helpful in understanding more about ADHD:

- **Rapid rise in people being diagnosed:** Based on a health records analysis by a commercial data-gathering company, *Time* reported that "more adults ages 22 to 44 sought care for ADHD in 2021 versus 2020, and . . . 15% more adults in this age group had an Adderall prescription in the middle of 2021 compared to a year earlier." Moreover, "almost twice as many women ages 23 to 49 got new ADHD diagnoses from 2020 to 2022, and . . . diagnostic rates have also risen among girls in recent years. People of color are also being diagnosed more frequently."[4]

- **Some reasons for this large increase:** Today there is more awareness, more and better diagnostic tools, and less stigma about giving prescription medications to children. As a result, we are only now discovering the full extent of the condition. Another reason may be that the ease of obtaining a diagnosis has been linked to the availability of competitive medications.* An article in the *Journal of Attention Disorders*, titled "Sudden Increases in U.S. Stimulant Prescribing: Alarming or Not?" concluded, "We cannot be certain that all patients prescribed stimulants have ADHD or that all prescriptions represent appropriate or effective treatment."[5]

- **ADHD is difficult to diagnose:** Childhood and adult issues of anxiety and hyperactivity can have many other causes. Unfortunately, there has been a recent surge in people receiving the diagnosis without the suggested lengthy and expensive diagnostic analysis.

- **ADHD diagnosis means easy access to amphetamines:** A BBC documentary looking at the rise in ADHD prescriptions "sparked debate for suggesting that ADHD assessments undertaken at private clinics are 'rushed' and 'unreliable.' An

---

*There are more than forty different medications available to treat ADHD. Between 2010 and 2015, sales of ADHD medications increased from $7.9 billion to $11.2 billion in the US.

undercover reporter working for the BBC underwent assessments at three private clinics, each of which diagnosed him with [ADHD]. . . . But he was found not to have the condition after undergoing a 'more detailed, in-person NHS assessment."[6] Similarly, the 2018 Netflix documentary *Take Your Pills*[7] showcased the extensive use of Adderall by students in a middle-sized liberal arts college. Students who faked ADHD symptoms to get a diagnosis easily obtained amphetamine prescriptions.

- **Parental support for keeping students on medication:** A psychiatrist friend of Jim's took a job at a prestigious college. Upon reviewing medical charts of a number of freshmen, he discovered they were no longer showing signs of ADD or ADHD, for which they were still on meds. When he notified the parents of the good news that their children no longer needed meds, he almost lost his job. Parents told him in no uncertain terms that their children got into that school because of the performance-enhancing effects of the ADD/ADHD meds and that if he tried to take them off these meds, they would get him removed.

Whatever the medical issue, concern, or challenge, microdosing appears to improve voluntary control of one's emotional life, with greater intellectual focus and diminished physical symptoms, either for ADHD symptoms directly, or for mitigating the negative effects of prescription ADHD medications.

ADHD in Children

My six-year-old's teacher says my child has ADHD. My pediatrician says that while it's okay to medicate her, there are side effects, and she may be on the medication for many years. Is she too young to try microdosing?

The US government considers ADHD to be "one of the most common neurodevelopmental disorders of childhood. It is usually first diagnosed in childhood and often lasts into adulthood. Children with ADHD may have trouble paying attention, controlling impulsive behaviors (may act without thinking about what the result will be), or be overly active."[8]

While ADHD used to be considered a childhood condition that naturally disappeared with maturation, that is no longer the case. Psychiatrists now believe that treated or not, for many people, its effects last well past childhood. The official advice is to treat a child as soon as possible, even younger than age three. Unfortunately, however, most ADHD medications (even for the youngest of children) are stimulants.

The mechanism is not well understood, but for children with ADHD, who are often too agitated to do their schoolwork, these medications provide an increased capacity to focus and consciously control their behavior. For other characteristics of stimulants, including how they affect appetite and sleep, the impact is similar to how adults react. As one study put it, "Stimulants can offer substantial benefits for persons with ADHD, but also pose potential harms, including adverse effects, medication interactions, diversion and misuse, and overdoses."[9] Inappropriate diagnosis can lead to further unnecessary medications and other problems.

Another reason for the rise in individuals taking ADHD prescription medications at every age—one not discussed in the clinical literature—is that in July 2016, *the US government declared ADHD a disability.* "The U.S. Department of Education has issued guidelines aimed at preventing schools from discriminating against the growing numbers of students with [ADHD]. In a letter to school districts and a 'know your rights' document to be posted on its website . . . the department said schools must obey existing civil rights law to identify students with the disorder and **provide them with accommodations** to help them learn."[10] [Emphasis ours.]

In practice, what this means is that any student with an ADHD diagnosis must be given appropriate support and accommodations. Students (kindergarten through graduate school) with ADHD may be given more time to complete examinations, may only have to answer every other question on homework assignments, and may be allowed to use otherwise forbidden technology to assist with tasks. They also may be allowed breaks or time to move around, and be provided a separate room, free of distractions, for exams.

We asked a special education teacher, "If a student is well medicated, and still can request all that extra support, might they have a definite advantage over students without the diagnosis or the treatment?" Her response: "Most definitely, which is why parents are so eager to get those accommodations for their children. Who wouldn't want more time on tests?"

In 2017, According to the Total Patient Tracker (TPT) Database, of the more than 9.5 million people in the US taking ADHD drugs, 80,000 were under five.[11]

As for microdosing for young children, we are always hesitant about any interventions that can change brain chemistry during childhood. Although this is also the general medical opinion, for ADHD there seems to be remarkably little hesitation in recommending daily or even twice daily stimulants throughout childhood and beyond.

Mostly extrapolating from adults, it seems likely that microdosing will have fewer negative effects than current ADHD medications. While we have very few reports of microdosing's effectiveness in young children, if you are considering a prescription stimulant regimen or microdosing for a young child with ADHD, it makes sense to consult with a microdosing-informed physician or coach experienced with children.

ADHD–Duration of Benefits

Do people need to keep microdosing to get the same kind of attention span and other benefits that amphetamine meds give?

Microdoses are different from the medications they sometimes replace because so many medications are simply symptom suppressants. Amphetamines for ADHD make no pretense of improving the condition's underlying causes; they simply allow the person to function better.

Microdoses tend to allow the body to restore equilibrium so that symptoms lessen and eventually go away. Unfortunately, most researchers make little effort (and have no funding) to follow up on the participants in a study for very long. So while ADHD microdosing studies show clear improvements for participants, few long-term records exist.

What usually happens with microdosing is that as conditions improve, doses are lowered or taken less regularly, and then often stopped entirely. This is especially true for those who have been microdosing for a particular physical or mental health condition. However, those who have found their *overall* health has improved will keep microdoses on hand for other possible uses.

While there are few long-term records, it seems likely that ADHD will follow the general pattern. That is, after a certain level of improvement, there is likely to be a diminishment in microdosing, either by decreasing dosage or stopping entirely.

This pattern was partly confirmed by a friend of ours,* a microdosing coach who works with business executives with ADHD. With many of her clients, as their ADHD gets better†—supported both by taking microdoses and working with her in other ways (diet, exercise, breathwork)—they are able to taper down and get off their medications. As they continue to do well, their microdosing becomes more irregular, and eventually stops.

At some point in the future, however, some of their old symptoms may return. At this point, the tendency is for people to reflexively reach back to their old pharmaceutical medications.‡ But very quickly they

---

*Many thanks to Wendy Perkins Shoef, neuro-pleasure and ADHD coach.

†She also recommends a specific protocol for ADHD clients who are microdosing psilocybin: for business productivity purposes, it's best for them to take their dose at five or six p.m. *the day before* they want to have a focused productive day. She also suggests that sometime that evening they journal, or at least think about the next day for ten minutes, which psychologically primes them to take maximum advantage (starting in the morning) of the still-open microdosing window.

‡This reflexive reach-back makes sense if you put yourselves in the shoes of someone who is suddenly coming up against difficult symptoms that they thought were no longer part of their life. For such a person, it would be reasonable to think that even one dose of their pharmaceutical medication—which they know worked in the past—would probably work best to quickly extinguish those symptoms.

are reminded just how much they didn't like the undesired effects of the pharmaceutical in the first place, and return to microdosing.

This pattern probably holds for quite a few conditions. However, as discussed throughout, those who are microdosing for a specific condition and see widespread benefits elsewhere (such as better food choices, more exercise, less addictive behaviors, being more social), as well as those who experience increased wellness and enhanced abilities, will be less likely to completely stop their microdosing.

ADHD Medications

While most people prescribed ADHD medications are satisfied and grateful that their most serious symptoms are effectively suppressed, some individuals with ADHD may become interested in microdosing to alleviate ADHD symptoms or reduce the negative effects of ADHD medications.

Most of the prescribed medications are stimulants: Adderall, the best-known ADHD medication, is a combination of an amphetamine and dextroamphetamine, two central nervous system stimulants that can improve focus and reduce impulsivity by increasing dopamine and norepinephrine levels in the brain. As WebMD describes it: "Used to treat attention deficit hyperactivity disorder (ADHD). . . . It can help increase your ability to pay attention, stay focused on an activity, and control behavior problems. It may also help you to organize your tasks and improve listening skills."

There has been a rapid increase in the number of users in the last few years: There are over nine million people in the United States currently talking ADHD medications. According to the CDC, the number of adult women taking ADHD medications more than tripled from 2003 to 2015. And although women are generally more likely than men to be on prescription drugs, only half as many girls as boys take prescription ADHD medicines.

There are negative effects: While many adults say ADHD medications benefit them, published negative effects include nervousness, headaches, sleep problems, dizziness, dry mouth, vision changes, slowed speech, hoarseness, hallucinations, and even heart disease, high blood pressure, and seizures. You can also become addicted and experience withdrawal symptoms if you stop using it suddenly (Marc Myer interview, 2021). Caffeine, because it is also a stimulant, and alcohol, because people cannot accurately judge their level of intoxication, are contraindicated for anyone taking any ADHD medication.

Depression

Depression Generally

Does microdosing help depression?

Background: Depression is characterized by persistent feelings of gloom and a loss of interest in almost all aspects of social and work life. It affects how you feel, think, and behave. It is not sadness or grief, or feelings about a personal loss or difficulty. Depression is not about anything in particular; it can be and often feels pervasive. We know less about depression than you might think.

More people microdose for depression than for any other condition. Already the number one mental illness worldwide, depression massively increased during the pandemic. Dozens of medications are classified as antidepressants, with the best known being SSRIs (selective serotonin reuptake inhibitors). However, for a significant percentage of people, antidepressants don't work at all, and for many others, the negative effects outweigh the benefits. (See box on pages 123–124.)

The best known and most widely publicized high-dose studies showcase the benefits of psychedelics in alleviating depression, at least for a while. Remission can last for a month, or as long as a year, or even longer. However, with psychedelics still not being widely legally available, even some of the subjects in successful studies eventually find themselves looking for help again.*

An early study reported on those self-identifying as depressed, with almost all having failed to benefit from prior antidepressant medications or treatments. They all microdosed on the same protocol, and close to 80 percent rated themselves as highly improved (Fadiman and Korb, 2019).

The clearest description of the symptoms and their alleviation came to us from a twenty-six-year-old woman with a diagnosis of depression and no prior history. She had been to a psychiatrist prior to microdosing, then had spoken to friends who were taking prescription medications. She concluded that such medications were not sufficiently effective, and decided to look for alternatives.

Specifically, the key phrases she heard from her friends on medications were "loss of emotions, 'zombified,' lower or no sex drive, addiction to said drug," as well as other things she "found scary and disagreeable." After obtaining some psilocybin capsules from a friend, she wrote the following:

> "I was very cynical on whether or not this would actually work. But after about 30 mins I felt like a weight was slowly lifting off my shoulders . . . after the first capsule, I felt like my old self was inching back into view.
>
> After a couple weeks of dosing I started really enjoying being around people and socializing again, which I hadn't felt

---

*After a small and reportedly successful study in England, two of the participants sought us out a few months later desperate for help. They were advised about microdosing, but as this was before coaching, they got no more help than that. One reported complete remission and intended to continue microdosing as needed. The other reported on its benefit.

for a year or two. And I slowly stopped using food as a comfort, and lost some weight (without even trying) which was amazing as that was a part of my guilt and depression cycle.

Overall, the effects were very subtle; if someone had slipped these pills into my morning smoothie I would definitely not have guessed "oh something was in that." I would have just thought that I was having some really amazing days, and I was in a great mood all the time. So definitely small differences, but over time have made big differences in my life!"

She provided a summary table:

Problems I felt I had *before* microdosing	How I felt *after* the first 3 weeks
Feelings of hopelessness	Overall sense of peace
Low energy all the time	Stopped grinding my teeth
Social anxiety	Less headaches
Irritability	Less irritated with loved ones
TMJ	Higher sex drive (enjoying sex again)
Eating to make myself feel better	Feeling excited about things again
Stress	Enjoying self-care routines
Weight gain	Weight loss (unintentionally)
Canceling plans due to panic about going out	Feeling more engaged in conversations
Headaches more than 4 times a week, sometimes for 2–3 weeks in a row	Not using food for comfort anymore
Unmotivated to do basic things like clean, shower, brush my teeth, take care of my skin	Able to do things with more deliberation
Feeling like I'm only living to worry about what's going to happen next	Able to focus more on the moment at hand, not just be stressing about what's coming
Feeling numb and like I don't really care about stuff, anything, anymore	Enjoying seeing friends and socializing again
Only being able to socialize if I drank	Able to socialize and have fun without drinking

Feeling depressed after drinking (even a glass of wine) Reduced sex drive Unable to be silent (without distraction of TV, phone, podcast) Spending the majority of my time in bed or on the sofa Avoiding friends and loved ones	Able to enjoy moments without my phone, TV, or some sort of distraction Want/need to be outside more and to have more experiences in general

Additional Reports

Depression is often a severe and debilitating condition, frequently leading to other conditions, especially when existing medications seem ineffective or have negative effects that are debilitating in themselves. The next reports exemplify some of these issues.

- [Twenty-nine-year old Canadian woman] "In the midst of this last severely depressed episode (the worst parts lasting approximately 2 years) along with my usual holistic therapies I started microdosing with mushrooms. The results astounded me. Within days I was feeling more than I had in years. I felt joy and beauty in pure and simple ways as I had not been able to for years.

   The ability to FEEL those things was what truly floored me. I had been able to see and, even on some level, appreciate good and positive and beautiful things even in the depths of my despair and apathy, but to be able to FEEL them was something I had lost the ability to do. . . . The benefits I experienced from my self-medication with psilocybin were far more effective than any legal drug. Not to mention I experienced essentially no negative side effects."

- "I'm a 30-year-old male. Lifelong journey with addictions, depression, and crippling anxiety. Three months of microdosing has changed the ******* game. I love myself unlike how I have ever loved myself before."

- "I am overall lighter and everyday things feel easier. Showers felt so hard. Cooking felt hard, taking the dog outside felt hard. I can do these things with no problem now. I even cleaned my whole place this weekend. I had an exceptionally stressful few weeks at work and I dove in head-first instead of hiding in bed with french fries crying. I have a vision for my future and two months ago didn't even want to live into the future."

- "I started my microdosing journey at the start of the year because I was feeling hopeless with the numerous amounts of medication I was taking for bipolar two. I've done ketamine trials with great success, but it wore off after a year, and I started on a downward spiral again.

  Microdosing every other day now and suicidal thoughts have become non-existent again. I feel comfortable enough to stop taking Trintellix [vortioxetine] and Rexulti [brexpiprazole]. Even the Valium I thought I needed I don't want to take anymore (been on benzos for eight years). Life changing medicine this is."

- [Parent describing a senior in a Dutch high school] "Even though he likes his new school, he has troubles with getting up in the morning and being late to school.

  After starting microdosing, it changed EVERYTHING. He went back to being this sweet and loving kid. He smiles, truly feels happy, hasn't been late to school since, and is getting up in the morning without issues. He is connecting to us, having conversations, interacting over dinner (something that never happened before), and takes responsibility for his actions. He even has a girlfriend now, who he brought home a few times (in the past his personal life was a mystery to us; he would NEVER say names of his friends, let alone bring them to the house).

  He is studying and taking school seriously. He still has problems with concentration, but it is getting better. Last week he had a test week, and he literally spent all night preparing for the tests (never happened before). We started visiting open days in universities (Leiden, TU Delft, UVA . . . he wants to study data analysis and AI). It was a hard and bumpy ride to get where we are, but without the truffles it would have not happened."

Different Effects of Microdoses and Antidepressants

Depression has been of great interest since the start of modern microdosing research. Jim recalls:

> Soon after Sophia Korb and I began working together, we set up a website, microdosingpsychedelics.com, with basic information about substances, doses, and the original protocol (one day dose, two days with no dose). We explained that we were gathering information about people's experiences, and that anything we learned would be added to this site, so it would be more helpful to others. We asked people to fill out a daily mood list (PANAS)[12] of positive and negative feelings, take daily notes on anything they noticed, and at the end of a month send us a report of what they had learned. Many of those early reports are in this book.

PANAS stands for "Positive and Negative Affect Schedule." It lists twenty emotional states, ten positive and ten negative:

Positive: interested, excited, strong, enthusiastic, proud, alert, inspired, determined, attentive, active
Negative: distressed, upset, guilty, scared, hostile, irritable, ashamed, nervous, jittery, afraid*

Each day people checked off how strongly they'd felt each emotion: "Very slightly or not at all/a little/moderately/quite a bit/extremely."

---

*Jim worried that the differences between some of the words—like "scared" and "afraid"—were almost non-existent. Sophia said that if we used this widely accepted test in our research, no one would ever question it. She was correct.

When we analyzed several hundred reports from people who'd said they were depressed and then microdosed, we found that negative feelings declined, week by week, and positive feelings strengthened each week.

Based on our own results from that initial data gathering and the results of other microdosing organizations and coaches, we have come to understand that microdoses and effective antidepressants are not equivalent.

SSRIs, when they are effective, soften the impact of negative emotions. People report that they are much more able to deal with difficult situations and feelings because they are less painful and disruptive. In many cases, they report they no longer feel some of those emotions at all.

Many reports about negative emotions are similar: "My upsets are less upsetting. Things still go wrong, but I'm able just to deal with them not to be incapacitated." "I'm no longer having suicidal thoughts." "I have down days, but now I'm more likely to be *pissed off* and do something about it rather than collapse in self-pity."

The major difference appears to be *that those who are microdosing almost always describe an upsurge in happiness—an increased ability to feel pleasure and enjoy other people.* They have renewed positive feelings about their lives overall. Antidepressants might be described more accurately as "emotional suppressants" in that one feels less bad, but also has reduced feelings overall.

A common major complaint about antidepressants—even from people reporting far less depression—is diminished happiness. Perhaps this is too simple, but it's generally accurate to say that:

> SSRIs make one's world less bad;
> Microdosing makes one's world less bad and more glad.

Recognizing this fundamental difference makes it easier to see how individuals who microdose for depression are not only shaking themselves loose from that depression but also discovering—and for many, it is a revelation—*that they can actually be happy,* independent of external events.

First Study Specifically Designed for Microdosing

The first depression study specifically designed with a microdosing proto-col in mind notes two obstacles that have limited formal clinical research for specific conditions. The first, discussed elsewhere, is the high cost of monitoring any long-term study. The second is the almost universal study feature of fixed doses from onset to completion. Microdosing, on the other hand, ideally begins with a low dose—guessed to be below any noticeable effect—then is raised slowly until the optimum dose (the sweet spot) is reached. After that, especially for physical or mental condi-tions, it is often reduced gradually until discontinued.

Undertaken by a group of microdosing-informed clinicians, the study was "the first reported case on the suspension of conventional pharma-cological treatment in conjunction with treatment with microdoses of psilocybin."[13] The subject, with a long prior history of mental issues, in-cluding one hospitalization, was "a 19-year-old nonbinary patient diag-nosed with major depressive disorder. . . . Assessed weekly over 7 months using clinical history, laboratory tests and the validated Hamilton De-pression Scale. [The scale is 1–17, 0–7 is normal range, subject at onset scored 9.] A complete symptomatic remission was observed, and a sus-pension of conventional pharmacological treatment with improvements in communication, social interaction and general well-being."[14]

The patient had been in treatment for two years with antidepres-sants and antipsychotics. Prior to microdosing, the patient was taking 100 milligrams of sertraline and 125 micrograms of quetiapine. Over the next two months, the quetiapine was reduced and finally discontin-ued. "Subsequently a progressive decrease in sertraline was started until its suspension, with no symptoms of discontinuation being evident. The dose of the mushroom was reduced and it was completely discon-tinued after an additional month: No alterations were observed in the clinical laboratory and the Hamilton scale value was 0. The patient was able to function in recreational spaces with ingenuity and enthusiasm, achieved a more demanding and complex job change, and became independent from his family of origin along with his partner. He was able to sustain this with efficiency and responsibility."[15]

Depression: The Truth Is, We Don't Know Very Much

Depression, regardless of what you may have been told or read, is not well understood. It cannot be physically measured, either in the blood or the brain. It's not a chemical imbalance in the brain, and it can't be cured by tweaking brain chemistry.

There are diverse methods for measuring depression, mostly questionnaires. Psychologist Eiko Fried identified seven popular scales that included a total of 125 questions and encompassed fifty-two disparate symptoms. Forty percent of the symptoms appeared in only a single scale, and the only symptom captured on all scales was "sad mood."[16] As Fried later put it in an interview, current ways of measurement "leave you with a really impoverished, tiny look."[17]

It's hard to treat what you can't measure or even barely begin to describe. Fried concludes: "Without good measurements, how can you possibly diagnose depression, determine whether symptoms get better with treatments or even prevent it in the first place?"[18]

What About Serotonin?

Since the 1960s, we have all been told about the "serotonin hypothesis." ("Hypothesis" is a scientific term for a guess.) According to Moncrieff and Horowitz:

Although first proposed in the 1960s, the serotonin theory of depression started to be widely promoted by the pharmaceutical industry in the 1990s in association with its efforts to market a new range of antidepressants, known as selective serotonin-reuptake inhibitors or SSRIs. The idea was also endorsed by official institutions such as the American Psychiatric

Association, which still tells the public that "differences in certain chemicals in the brain may contribute to symptoms of depression." In the period of this marketing push, antidepressant use climbed dramatically, and they are now prescribed to one in six of the adult population in England.[19]

It is true that antidepressants affect levels of serotonin in the brain. However, a comprehensive 2022 study published in *Molecular Psychiatry* finds no consistent data supporting the idea that low serotonin causes depression. As one article commented, "After decades of study, there remains no clear evidence that serotonin levels or serotonin activity are responsible for depression."[20]

Drugs that increase brain serotonin levels do ease the depression symptoms of as many as half of those who take them. However, this doesn't mean that depression was *caused* by serotonin. As Nassir Ghaemi, MD, wrote in *Psychology Today* in 2022, "That's backward logic."[21] (Consider: aspirin can ease a headache, but a headache is not caused by low aspirin.) Or as Moncrieff and Horowitz write, "There are other explanations for antidepressants' effects. In fact, drug trials show that antidepressants are barely distinguishable from a placebo (dummy pill) when it comes to treating depression."[22] As Alina Cristea concludes with regard to previous research, "Reducing depression to specific problems in biology in the brain didn't work."[23]

The Downsides of SSRIs

This book includes many stories of those hoping to taper off pharmaceuticals. Why? In addition to "fixing" something (low serotonin) that the evidence does not indicate is a problem, SSRIs and other antidepressants cause a wide variety of negative effects.

According to Jakobsen and Kirsch, "Antidepressants seem to have minimal beneficial effects on depressive symptoms and increase the risk of both serious and non-serious adverse events" (2020). Sansone and Sansone add that "[SSRI] exposure has been occasionally associated with both behavioral apathy and emotional blunting. While frequently described as separate entities, these two syndromes are mutually characterized by indifference" (2010).

Moncrieff and Horowitz conclude that "if antidepressants exert their effects as placebos, or by numbing emotions, then it is not clear that they do more good than harm.... [W]e do not understand what temporarily elevating serotonin or other biochemical changes produced by antidepressants do to the brain. **We conclude that it is impossible to say that taking SSRI antidepressants is worthwhile, or even completely safe**" (2022; emphasis added).

Remember, however, if you're taking antidepressants, it's very important you don't stop (or substantially change what you're taking) without obtaining and following your doctor's instructions for doing so safely.

Among the reasons this brain chemistry approach has not led to effective treatment is its neglect of the impact of external events. Fatigue, as an obvious example, plays an important role in depression. A recent study of first-year doctors in the US, published in the *New England Journal of Medicine,* found that "the more these doctors worked, the higher the rate of depression," as was true for healthcare workers in emergency departments during the pandemic.[24] Real world events matter.

Science writer Laura Sanders[25] sums all this up: "We will never have a simple explanation for depression; we are now learning that one cannot possibly exist."[26]

Why, then, have high doses (in psychedelic-assisted psychother-apy and with individuals using them on their own), as well as mi-crodoses, been so successful? Perhaps it is because with psychedelics the entire system experiences increased flexibility, reduced inflam-mation, a return to a healthy equilibrium, and increased neuroplas-ticity. This overall physical-mental tune-up is likely at the heart of most improvements.

A Game Changer! Literally a week before this book's typesetting was finished, a report came in from MindBio Therapeutics on their Canadian Phase 2A clinical trial of eight weeks of at-home LSD mi-crodosing for depression. Three months later, patients still sustained a 62.8 percent reduction in depression symptoms. This proof of concept of a clinically successful study correlates with the numerous real-world detailed individual reports included here. The company suggests that microdosing could be a "globally scalable, effective, affordable way to treat patients" (MindBio Therapeutics, 2024). We agree.

Long COVID

Can microdosing help decrease or eliminate any of the symptoms of long COVID?

Long COVID is not COVID; it is an umbrella term covering the aftereffects of COVID that last well after the virus itself is no longer present. As *Time* puts it:

> Long Covid, a chronic condition that affects millions of
> people who've had COVID-19, often looks nothing like acute
> COVID-19. Sufferers report more than 200 symptoms affect-
> ing nearly every part of the body, including the neurologic,
> cardiovascular, respiratory, and gastrointestinal systems. The
> conditions range in severity but many so-called "long-haulers"

are unable to work, go to school, or leave their homes with any sort of consistency.[27]

Long COVID Reports

Here are five reports. The first is from an executive at a psychedelic startup, the second from Reddit, the third from *Time* (whose health correspondent Jamie Ducharme has written a series of COVID-related articles). The fourth—unusual for this book—is a high-dose report (also from *Time*), and the last is from a family friend of Jim's wife.

REPORT 1

"I thought I was recovering fine from a light case of COVID. When I began to feel less and less well, I just put it off. What woke me up was when my physician said that I should see a speech therapist because my speech was getting so slurred that it was hard to understand. I realized that I had stopped microdosing some months earlier and returned to my usual dose and protocol. My speech normalized and my fatigue as well within a few weeks."

REPORT 2

"I had long COVID for four months which included migraines every day, and of course the fatigue and weariness. I saw no light at the end of the tunnel. I tried microdosing .2g every 3rd day for a month, the normal routine. Within a week, I felt almost free of all of my symptoms. Ever since, I have been free of my symptoms."

REPORT 3

Renee, age fifty-three: After a suspected case of COVID-19 in 2020 left her with a loss of smell, a rapid heart rate, dizziness, ringing in her ears, brain fog, psychosis, hallucinations, and suicidal thoughts, she decided to try microdosing . . . taking small amounts of LSD every few days for a month.

She says, "I started to feel connected to humanity again. I had emotions again. I had some joy again. I felt normal." Her cognitive functioning improved dramatically, and she felt her creativity come back.

REPORT 4

[A megadose usually has an entirely different range of effects, but at least in this instance, there was a similar outcome.]

A woman, age thirty-one, after a year of long COVID, was still "short of breath, tired, and riddled with heart, motor, cognitive, gastrointestinal, and menstrual issues." Having had prior psychedelic experience, she gave herself five grams of mushrooms. "She woke up the next morning with a normal heart rate, breathing more freely than she had in a long time. After that, her period stabilized and her brain fog and motor dysfunction cleared. She got her energy back. She still has a few lingering symptoms."[28]

REPORT 5

This is a report of a very severe long-term COVID case that responded to microdosing a few years after the young man first had COVID. He is still far from recovered. This is a summary of reports sent to Jim by the boy's mother.

In early 2020, thirteen-year-old "Daniel" was a successful popular 9th grader. He was athletic, at the top of the class academically, a social leader, popular, and had just started seeing his first girlfriend.

January 2020: He was admitted to the ER with a fever spiking over 105, delirium, severe exhaustion, and extreme pain, and had coughed up blood. Although he was cared for by ER staff in hazmat suits, he was diagnosed as having the flu and sent home.

School, learning, sports, friends, going anywhere, doing anything—they all became too much to physically bear.

Slowly, he began to recover. Slowly he worked toward recovery, though unable to regain energy and strength.

December 2020, he was reinfected. Symptoms included low oxygen levels, inability to concentrate or complete mental tasks, panic attacks, brain fog, memory issues, and excruciating pain to the point where he would be in bed in a fetal position screaming "Mom! Make it stop!" The feeling of knives in his stomach any time he ate or drank led to severe weight loss.

Many hospitals, many doctors. No help. Because of COVID-induced inflammation, he developed median arcuate ligament syndrome (MALS), finally relieved by laparoscopic surgery, after which he was able to eat and began to regain weight. He also had heart damage and several other physical issues. His condition stabilized with him on eight medications.

Later, stem cell therapy initially showed initial promise of remarkable improvements. After the first infusion, he walked for four miles up and down hills and was not sore or tired the next day, but for only the initial dose. Six weeks of intermittent stem cell treatment followed. It is likely that stem cells reduced viral load and helped build cells in his brain, heart, etc. Overall, however, no major changes after stem cells began, beyond a slight up-leveling of function.

Stable at home with hyperbaric oxygen treatment, once a week for seven months, then four times a week for four months for over a year. Stellate ganglion blocks [nerve injections] increased energy somewhat. However, depression, anxiety, and lack of social energy remained. Brain and memory function stayed low.

Microdosing started in 2023: Using psilocybin and functional mushroom mix, following the Fadiman protocol. From his mother's report, after one month:

"Depression—gone, vanished, lifted
Anxiety—gone, vanished, lifted
Social energy—from unwilling to be with any family to full participation in family activities and holiday gatherings
Energy—still low. Needing to plan for any event, including rest, but able to do so.
Sense of humor—returned
Allowed touch and eye contact, hugs, snuggle with pets
Memory and intelligence—back to pre-COVID levels
Self-care—showering, shaving, haircuts, all had been too much before microdosing"

Myofascial, muscular, nerve, and bone pain all decreased tremendously, allowing for greater physical functioning. In his mother's words:

"He is limited by long COVID and the existing disorders of POTS, hEDS, CFS/ME & MCAD, but his spirit, desire, and ability to function in life and look to the future have returned substantially with microdosing.

Microdosing eliminated three years of depression in four weeks. Brought back motivation, zest for life, eliminated pain and brain fog, brought back socialization, eliminated anxiety, and improved sleep. Schoolwork is easier, interacting is easier, thinking is easier. Light has returned to his eyes. His humor is back to a delightful degree. His ease of being, compassion, and desire for touch and interaction are all back."

According to Daniel himself, "The most important of all the things [treatments] I have done has been the mushrooms."

Today, vaccinations are working better and better, and Paxlovid, taken immediately after a positive test, protects many from their infection becoming more serious. However, recovery from long COVID "remains rare."[29] Different surveys report different recovery rates, but none show more than a 20 percent full recovery rate, and even those individuals are predicted to be at increased risk for related health problems for years.

"As of now, there is no one-size-fits-all treatment for long COVID, nor any treatment guaranteed to work at all."[30] There are no clinical research studies testing psychedelics, but with the cases cited here and ones showing equal or greater improvement, psychedelics are beginning to get serious medical attention as one more possible way to help the millions of people afflicted by long COVID.

Daniel's family asked us to append the following note, specifically to alert individuals with long COVID and their medical support:

> Long COVID sufferers often wind up with HPOTS (hyperadrenergic postural orthostatic tachycardia syndrome), hEDS (hypermobile Ehlers-Danlos syndrome), ME/CFS (myalgic encephalomyelitis/chronic fatigue syndrome), and/or MCAS (mast cell activation syndrome).[31] Anytime we speak of long COVID, if we include the triggered disorders, we help shorten the search for help that can save so much pain, and likely permanent damage, even lives.

Microdosing Along With and Tapering Off Medications

Can I stop my meds and switch to microdosing? Or do I need to be off the meds before I start?

One major reason people microdose is to help them come off medication that is no longer helpful, or whose negative effects have come to overshadow its benefits.

You may never have read one, but you get a tiny packet of detailed information with every prescription of medication. Along with an unnerving list of known side effects, there is often a description of potential problems should you miss a dose—even a single dose—of the medication.

Stopping an SSRI cold turkey, for example, may bring on a deeply depressed mental state, accompanied by "suicidal ideation" (actively thinking about the possibility of suicide).

For your own safety, the approved medical alternative to stopping completely is "tapering" (also called "tapering off"). Tapering involves reducing the dose of the medication slowly and carefully, often over a period of weeks or months, until stopping it no longer puts you at risk. If you wish to taper off a medication and begin microdosing, you need to work with the healthcare professional or organization who writes your prescriptions. Ask for their help, advice, and scheduling suggestions. Depending on their openness and understanding of microdosing, you can let them know that you will be microdosing to support the tapering process.

What we've been told, over and over, is that tapering was easier with microdosing and happened more quickly. There were even reports from those who had previously failed to come off their medications and finally succeeded when microdosing was added to their tapering regimen. As for the second question—should you be off a medication before beginning microdosing—while it may be better to first stop a medication, the reality is that many people on many kinds of medications start microdosing before tapering them. However, even if you feel better quickly—as is common with depression, for example—continue the tapering schedule laid out by your practitioner for at least a few more weeks. If you continue to feel no need for the medication, then you may taper down more quickly, but do not abruptly stop tapering.

Once you are safely off the medication, you can test whether a smaller microdose is more appropriate. Often, without any conscious intention, people find their general health improving, with shifts in diet, improved sleep, additional exercise or meditation, and reduced consumption of alcohol, tobacco, coffee, and cannabis. Microdosing apparently eases tapering, in part, because it helps bring the body and all its systems back into a healthier equilibrium.

Pain

Can microdosing help with long-term chronic pain?

Microdosing can indeed help with chronic pain.* (For specific conditions, see entries for migraine headaches, cluster headaches, traumatic brain injury, and shingles.)

Pain is not a choice. It is a consequence. It is blame-free. Even when caused by bad judgment, it is always unintended. Short-term pain is the body's way of preventing more pain or damage by stopping you from doing whatever you're doing.

Chronic pain is different.†

Researchers estimate that close to fifty million adults in the United States alone live with some degree of chronic pain. Most medications and procedures that lessen pain also have serious negative effects. Microdosing not only reduces pain but improves overall functioning. By lowering the incidence and severity of felt pain, it accelerates organic systemic healing.

Two recent studies have investigated the effects of microdosing on pain. One measured awareness of pain; the other compared the effectiveness of pain medications (opiates, ketamine, cannabis, and others) to psychedelic microdoses and macrodoses over a range of conditions.

The first study (Ramaekers et al., 2020) tested if a low dose of

---

*Pain is physical suffering or discomfort caused by illness or injury. Pain "is an unpleasant feeling, such as a prick, tingle, sting, burn, or ache. Pain may be sharp or dull. It may come and go, or it may be constant. You may feel pain in one area of your body, such as your back, abdomen, chest, pelvis, or you may feel pain all over" (Medline Plus, 2018, "Pain").

†"Chronic pain," as defined by Johns Hopkins Medicine, is "long-standing pain that persists beyond the usual recovery period or occurs along with a chronic health condition, such as arthritis. Chronic pain may be 'on' and 'off' or continuous. It may affect people to the point that they can't work, eat properly, take part in physical activity, or enjoy life" (Johns Hopkins Medicine, "Chronic Pain," n.d.).

LSD would affect pain perception in healthy volunteers. Subjects were given either five, ten, or twenty micrograms of LSD. The magnitude of the effect was similar to "the same test with opioids, such as oxycodone 20 mg and morphine 10–20 mg." As we have seen, since microdosing improves functioning, it's no surprise that this study found that those who were microdosing were better able to tolerate pain for a few minutes.

The second study (Bonnelle et al., 2022) was an investigation of the actual experience of chronic pain sufferers who had microdosed and macrodosed to lessen their pain. "We report the results . . . from individuals suffering with chronic pain and who have [prior] . . . experience with psychedelics."[32] The survey compared analgesic effects from macrodoses, microdoses, and conventional medications on a number of dimensions. Any respondent who reported any level of relief at any dose of any psychedelic was asked to determine changes in:

- Pain intensity
- Pain acceptance
- Pain interference with daily activities
- Pain-induced emotional distress
- Duration of pain relief

In addition, they "were asked to compare the level of pain reduction achieved with the most effective psychedelic compound to that of the most effective conventional pain medication (including cannabis)."[33]

The respondents had sixteen different kinds of pain. In order, the most common types were back pain, joint pain, tendon and ligament pain, arthritis, and migraine headache pain.

The results: "Macrodosing and microdosing were both associated with perceived improvements in pain intensity, acceptance of pain, interference caused by pain and emotional stress." While macrodoses of psychedelics were more effective than microdoses, both were significantly more effective than NSAIDs, opioids, or cannabis.

Focus and intention apparently mattered, as people who micro-dosed expressly for pain reported more pain relief than people who microdosed for other reasons.

Pain Reports

As a senior researcher in a major medical school once said, "The problem with data is it does not give us a real picture of any individual." Let's consider reports from our own database.

REPORT 1

About five years ago, a report came in that was sufficiently remarkable that Jim contacted the man and interviewed him for over an hour. More than twenty years earlier, a large piece of mechanical equipment had fallen on him and broken his back just below his neck and just above his sacrum. He was told by his medical team that there was an operation that might repair the damage, but that it was not guaranteed.

"What will be the result if the operation is not successful?"

"You would not be able to walk ever again, but you will have less pain."

Declining the operation, he looked for alternatives. He found a pain management expert—a medical doctor and a professor at an Ivy League university. Put on opiates, he was carefully monitored. He recovered enough to return to work using opiates to keep his pain under control. Over the next twenty years, he continued to work at jobs demanding both strength and endurance. He did not exceed the prescribed dose or protocol, and had none of the problems associated with many opiate patients.

In the twentieth year of his treatment, the federal government issued new regulations to the medical profession as part of their attempt to grapple with growing opiate overuse. The professor told him that the new regulations prevented him from continuing to correctly prescribe to his functioning pain patients. Unable to help these patients, he resigned his academic position and his medical affiliation. He moved to Ecuador, where he now has a commercial flower farm.

Devastated, the man sought out alternatives. Cannabis was sufficiently helpful that he no longer contemplated suicide, but he was still unable to function very well and remained in chronic pain. Eventually, he read about treating pain with microdoses of psilocybin.

He found that with microdosing he was able to do physical work again. When asked how he felt now, he said, "On days when I microdose, the pain is just a tingle. When I am unable to microdose, the pain is intolerable."

REPORT 2

(From a microdosing coach:) "My client is a 70-year-old contractor. Two years ago, he fell off a roof and broke bones all over his body. Today, mostly healed, he successfully uses microdosing to control his daily pain and is working again."

REPORT 3

A Canadian professional hockey player—like so many others—was forced to retire from hockey because of too many concussions. All the treatments recommended by his physicians and by several traumatic brain injury facilities failed. To minimize his throbbing head pain, he rarely left his darkened bedroom. After some months of microdosing, however, he was not only able to resume his life but recovered enough to become engaged and was recently married. He no longer feels any need to continue microdosing.

REPORT 4

A man injured in an automobile accident some years earlier reported that he was in constant pain and was hopeful that microdosing would allow him to use opiates less. After several weeks, he said, "On a scale of 1 to 10, my pain is about the same. However, I'm much less bothered by the pain; I feel somehow more distant from it. I'm less of a pain patient and more like someone who 'has a pain.'" Other reports have been similar in people stating that their pain has become more peripheral. Microdosing allows these individuals to distance themselves from their pain more successfully.

CONCLUSION

We've heard from people who microdose for chronic pain that their pain either lessened or, if it had the same intensity, was no longer as disturbing or central to their lives. People shifted from "being in pain" to "having pain." The pain took up less space in their consciousness and had less of an effect on their daily activities.

We don't know the full extent to which psychedelics can serve as an alternative to conventional pain medications. While there is justified hesitation in recommending high doses, it may be that microdoses, with their robust safety profile and low incidence of negative effects, may become a first-level medication of choice for chronic, palliative, and even cancer-related pain.

Research results and individual reports lead us to conclude that compared to taking conventional pain medications, microdosing psychedelics is a realistic and validated alternative.

A Pain-Free Lower Back

"A little while back I went in for a checkup. My numbers impressed the Dr. and she even mentioned I was not reapplying for my prescription of anti-inflammatory. She talked more about how positive the numbers were, and I reminded her she hadn't asked why I stopped using the anti-inflammatory, because 'degenerative disk disease doesn't get better.'

She said, 'Right, why aren't you using it?' I told her I hadn't needed it for over 3 years now because I had found something better.

She asked what it was because she also suffers from the same condition and practically lives on Ibuprofen. I told her it's microdosing. 'It's what?' I said it again and she asked me if I'd explain. She listened as I explained and wasn't aware of this practice or the research that's been done.

I sent her links and she contacted me wanting more info on how I started. She recently let me know it's working very well for her personally, as she has been painless and other meds-free for a week after several weeks of microdosing, and thanked me."

Women's Health

How does microdosing affect the health of women in particular, especially around issues like pregnancy, breastfeeding, and early parenting?

While we will briefly consider what the US government and the Microdosing Institute have to say here, this section on women's health will mostly focus on the real-world evidence[34] generously shared with us by Mikaela de la Myco, Naomi Tolson, and the Mothers of the Mushroom Project. Their first-ever survey on the effects of psychedelics during pregnancy and the postpartum period had about 400 responses—those who macrodosed, those who only microdosed (about 100, whose reports you see here), and those who did both.[35] It is a unique source of information about positive and negative results as well as real-world difficulties and challenges.

With full permission, we present a special section of representative responses to some of the questions in the full survey, and have also included some of Mikaela de la Myco's comments. More information about the results of the survey can be found at their website, mushwomb.love/mothersofthemushroom.

Pregnancy (During and After)

What's the official advice about whether it's safe to microdose when you're pregnant?

Although women of childbearing age have been taking psychedelics since the 1960s, the US government appears to have no information about their effect during or after pregnancy. The US National Institutes of Health "Fact Sheet" tells us there was one animal study and it did not find any increased chance of birth defects. The Microdosing Institute acknowledged that there was no official information but did include a summary of some indigenous perspectives:

> Consider the Shipibo-Conibo group of the Peruvian Amazon, who consume ayahuasca, and the Wixárika (Huichol) group in Mexico and Southern USA whose rituals involve sweat lodges and Peyote cactus. They both argue their rituals are harmless to unborn babies, and babies who receive their mother's milk, and to the contrary, there are many benefits for the baby and the mom alike. . . . Amongst the Shipibo, taking small doses of ayahuasca in ceremony while breastfeeding is common, across this culture, *curanderos* [healers] state that it supports both the mother and the baby and helps them to be even more in alignment with one another and with spirit. . . . After consulting with their shaman, some women intentionally consume plant medicines, in various doses, throughout the entirety of their pregnancy. Others wait until the first term has passed.[36]

The Institute concludes its indigenous historical walkabout with this caution:

> Regarding these traditional practices, we must also be aware that cultural context is important, and while there is clear evidence of safe psychedelic use during pregnancy and breastfeeding in other cultures, it does not imply that this information is directly applicable in non-traditional settings.[37]

Its final recommendation is also cautious:

> It is important to once again highlight that using any of the most common microdosing substances, LSD or psilocybin, during your pregnancy or while breastfeeding is still brand-new and un-researched territory in the West. However, **vast anecdotal evidence strongly suggests that microdosing can support one's mental health**, which we recognize can be a common struggle during the life shifts that occur during pregnancy and after. **Given the lack of scientific evidence, we cannot recommend for or against microdosing during pregnancy or breastfeeding.**[38] (Emphases added.)

Reports from Women

What benefits did you notice in your pregnancy?

- "Able to come back to my body rather than always being in my head."
- "A better outlook on my overall situation. My baby was far more active while dosing which lessened any anxiety I had. I enjoyed life more than when I wasn't on a dose."
- "I was present in my body; I was clear in my mind and able to regulate my emotions. I was able to separate my fear and anxiety. I was the best version of myself on low days."

- "Boost in energy and motivation to do everyday tasks amongst exhaustion and low mood."
- "Intuitive, relaxing, connected, centered."
- "I have the happiest baby."
- "I actually got pregnant [while microdosing]. We had struggled for years."
- "Pain relief, eased intense emotionality, deeper connection to my body, more clear mind, less concern about other people's ideas."
- "I felt more motivated, had greater capacity to cope with emotions and hormonal changes. I felt more relaxed and present."
- "Light, happy and motivated during what was a really hard time."
- "Years worth of suicidal thoughts disappeared in two microdoses."

Comment from Mikaela de la Myco: "Concerning early pregnancy and morning sickness, the women in the survey found that any morning sickness or nausea associated with the pregnancy was not really helped by microdosing mushrooms, and that instead, cannabis emerged as the preferred treatment method."

Microdosing While Breastfeeding

The earliest draft of this book looked briefly at microdosing while breastfeeding:

> We have no reports of microdosing having any effect on breastfeeding. . . . Psilocybin, eliminated through the kidneys, is mostly gone within three hours; LSD is metabolized by the liver and is almost completely excreted in between four and six hours.[39] To be conservative, when possible, breastfeed before, or several hours after, microdosing.

Since then, while microdosing's popularity has risen throughout all demographics—including breastfeeding mothers—no substantially different recommendations have emerged.

No research, no data, no advice.

While reminding us that there are no studies on microdosing while breastfeeding, the Microdosing Institute has posted some specific recommendations:

"Microdoses of psychedelic substances can be metabolized and excreted within twenty-four hours. Extrapolating this to a breastfeeding mother:

- Only use small doses, 100 mg/0.1 gram of psilocybin or less.
- Follow the Fadiman protocol of one day on, two days off (or even less frequently, such as microdosing twice a week).
- On non-microdosing days, pump milk enough to last twenty-four to thirty-six hours to utilize during microdosing days.
- For twenty-four hours after microdosing, pump and discard any milk produced during this period" ("Microdosing While Breastfeeding," Microdosing Institute).

Breastfeeding Benefits

Did you notice any benefits to a) yourself or b) to your baby, and what were the benefits when ingesting mushrooms while breastfeeding?

Most of these excerpts are from women who only microdosed. Most of the responses were about themselves, some about their child.

- "Way more present, creative, more empathic, more energy, better socially, my little one was livelier and more empathic. Totally went off coffee, which I'm normally addicted to. Minimal interest in alcohol. Already low but almost nonexistent when dosing."

- "I'm so much more relaxed. I don't rush around. I let things be. I feel my baby is getting a better version of myself. My baby is incredibly curious and brave."
- "I just felt so much more relaxed and connected and baby probably senses it too. I was in the process of weaning from breastfeeding. It made it easier for both of us as we took our time."
- "For myself, I was able to be more present and patient with my baby and less overwhelmed with her crying. She definitely benefited from my ability to be present with her."
- "While breastfeeding I noticed that my feelings of overwhelm and exhaustion were minimal. More patience with my son and an overall happy attitude."
- "It allowed me to slow down and be more present during long hours of breastfeeding, enjoying it at full capacity, not wanting to rush to get some things done."
- "Yes. Felt closer to baby and happier as a mom. I felt like I could connect to him more and my depression was lessened."
- "My son is hitting all of his milestones early and seems to be very happy and charismatic. He's always smiling and laughing."
- "I was apprehensive about microdosing while breastfeeding, but after the first time, seeing that it had no effect on him and noticing the benefits to me, I no longer questioned it. I noticed a calmer demeanor even though I was tired, I noticed that I felt peace in making decisions. I trusted my intuition more."
- "I was freed of postpartum anxiety almost instantly and felt less reactive in my mothering, less triggered and more spacious inside so that I could sit with the hard emotions of grieving the loss of self."

Breastfeeding Challenges

When specifically asked about breastfeeding *challenges* while microdosing, most of the women in the survey said there were none.

- "All benefits, no challenges."
- "I did not notice any challenges; it was blissful."
- "Not at all challenging to either me or my baby."
- "I haven't noticed any negatives to microdosing."

For a few women, there was a pattern of things getting worse before getting better, and some felt legal pressure or anxiety:

- "They [the mushrooms] challenged me to step up my game when things got hard. I.e.: helped me with my work on doing better."
- "We had a rough start to breastfeeding, and reclaiming that relationship once we were home was top priority. I didn't start microdosing untilv he was a few months old, but that was when my hormones were attempting to level out, him trying to figure out my fast letdown, all the intrusive thoughts from birth . . . ingesting mushrooms helped me gain clarity and grace with myself."
- "No challenges except legally."
- "Anxiety around getting my baby taken away if anyone found out. The great fear was losing my child through the government system."

Mikaela de la Myco noted that the majority of respondents (close to 75 percent) chose to consume mushrooms while breastfeeding, simply going forward with their normal breastfeeding routine and schedule. None of these women felt constrained by the conventional advice previously described.

For some respondents, "breastfeeding while microdosing made it a more comfortable and enjoyable experience." For others, because of the microdosing, the physical relationship and bond with the child became stronger, so *breastfeeding just went better overall,* from physical to emotional aspects. She concluded that most of her survey respondents had "positive experiences with breastfeeding while microdosing, however, some people felt it brought up things they had to process and deal with."

Parenting Benefits

What did you notice in your parenting that you attribute to the mushroom?

- "I was more in tune with my kiddo, more understanding with his growing."
- "The mushrooms gave me the ability to see beyond my current circumstance. I was able to react pragmatically to my baby instead of frantically, knowing that everything I was going through, each moment, was temporary."
- "More relaxed. More easygoing. Less hectic and rushed feeling. More pleasant emotions."
- "Calmer around screaming kids . . . easier to laugh and connect and appreciate my connection with my family."
- "A sense of complete calmness and peace, knowing that nothing is as serious as the world claims it to be. I find absolute joy in being a mama. I feel intimately connected with my child and the natural world, and am able to parent from a place of a larger sense of oneness with all."
- "I am much more present and connected to my daughter. I feel feelings of love throughout my body. I am able to be still with greater ease. I'm able to get on with the things I need to do more efficiently. Somehow I feel I have more hours in the day on my dosing days."
- "I notice that I move more slowly with my children, I don't rush as often from place to place. I take the time to notice what they are noticing. I am also able to more mindfully address inner child wounds and work on healing."

- "I was calmer, more patient and generally happier. I was less concerned about the dishes and more willing to go take a walk and spend quality time together."
- "I was more able to cope with the pressures of being a single mom; I was less stressed and less likely to fly off the handle."
- "I notice when I am upset and can catch myself before I dwell or lash out. I can question myself and have a second for reflection."
- "Oh my goodness so many things . . . I got my creative thinking back, my deep compassion and patience, I felt like I also could hear my intuition better . . . and because of that I was able to pick up on what my older kiddo was experiencing or subtle ways she was communicating. I found myself lingering in lovely tender moments with my girls . . . I was singing again, dancing, and just generally feeling lighter and more myself."

Parenting Challenges

What were the unwanted effects or challenges of ingesting mushrooms while parenting?

- "Anxiety [that] I was passing it to [my] baby."
- "I was tired when it wore off."
- "Sometimes dark and twisty stuff would come up. Intrusive thoughts. A heaviness sometimes accompanied the dose."
- "Getting the dose right. Initially it was too strong."
- "Probably the fact that since I'm doing it on my own as a solo parent, I don't have that sounding board if I'm doing things the right way. I've definitely become more conscious about not being biased from one viewpoint."
- "Feeling the need to keep it a secret for legal reasons while going through a custody battle."

- "I can't really have a drink while dosing, it messes up my sleep. Sometimes there can be a headache or most often a hard emotion that will be amplified on a dosing day."
- "The anxiety of accidentally taking 'too much.'"
- "A good regular reliable supplier."
- "Only challenges were trusting myself and the minimal information I could find that it was safe and wouldn't harm my baby."
- "The judgment from my midwives and judgment from other parents. Legality."

[The most common response was "none," and the most common challenge was "anxiety."]

Surprises

What surprised you about the mushroom journey?

- "That I didn't have to keep doing it. About two months in I noticed a mood change without needing my capsules."
- "I was surprised how long it took to really feel 'good' from taking them. I almost quit early on because of the burden I felt taking them at times, but the lightness I felt the next day kept me coming back."
- "How much better it worked than traditional pharmaceuticals and how quickly it worked!"
- "How confident I feel in this decision and how much changed in a highly positive way immediately."
- "All of the smacking benefits in such a small dose."
- "How normal I felt, how much more myself I felt. Less monkey mind. I worried I would be tripping but it was quite the opposite. Much more clarity and a positive mindset."
- "How quickly it lifted my suicidal thoughts. I mean after two doses that was gone."

- "How natural the effects felt. It's like the mushrooms dusted off all the equipment in my brain postpartum. How much I just felt like me but a better version. I wasn't 'altered,' I was centered."
- "That it seemed to help improve my milk supply, my connection with my baby, and overall environment."
- "That it was actually safe, that my intuition knew it would be safe and that there were many other parents on the same road as me."
- "That it was so subtle, almost unable to tell I had consumed them. But there's no denying I felt amazing from them."

Say to Others

What would you like to say to other mothers and pregnant/birthing people about your own experience?

- "Forming a relationship with mushrooms saved my life and allowed me to be the woman I've always aspired to be, always known I could be, with very few negative side effects."
- "I can't believe how well it works! I work in healthcare and feel like I was brainwashed by my pharmaceutical classes to ignore mushrooms."
- "If you want to support your nervous system, especially if you have had a few miscarriages or trauma during pregnancy or birth, I recommend it 100%."
- "MDing has brought a new calm to my world that didn't exist before. It's allowed me to move through my emotions and better communicate with my toddler and partner. It's created a beautiful opportunity for me to come back to nature and to myself as well."
- "You are not alone. You have an inner wisdom and knowing that will at times feel so far away you may doubt its existence."

- "There is a light at the end of the tunnel and it's mushrooms. You don't have to be medicated and turned into a zombie. You can feel everything and be ok. You can see your life for the beauty that it is and still have tough days. They settled me. They grounded me. They reminded me why I'm living and why I wanted to be a mama."

- "Mushrooms were the only thing that truly prepared me for birth and the transformation that comes with becoming a parent. It also gave me peace of mind that I was giving my baby the best possible start to life by microdosing mushrooms."

- "That mushrooms have and continue to make a positive difference. We can trust our plants! They are here for us, to help, to guide. For me it has really been being present with my baby and myself after this huge transition."

Recommend This Path?

Would you recommend this path to other people?

- "Yes, I would say it's far superior to antidepressants."
- "Wholeheartedly YES! Postpartum ritual should include work with these mushrooms. We will be better parents, partners, and people because of it."
- "Yes. Of course, it depends on a person's situation. But based on my experience I absolutely would."

[Almost every respondent answered "yes," "absolutely," "sure," "definitely," or something similar, with a few pointing out (wisely) that mushrooms will not be for everyone, and only individuals who feel called to microdosing during pregnancy should do so.]

Mikaela de la Myco's additional comments: A primary reason for abstaining from psilocybin during pregnancy, postpartum, and breastfeeding is due to the stigma faced by so many women, either internally or from their caregivers or community. However, for some women, "the reason to microdose is stronger than the possible negative outcome. The calling to ingest often comes from the need to rectify or repair something in their life that they don't want to pass down to their child, and they're willing to take the risk to be a well mother."[40]

Mikaela also noted that "most people recommended microdosing either saying they learned a lot from it, or that they're really grateful for it. Those who were seeking symptom relief in pregnancy did get the desired outcome they were looking for, or at least came close to that desired outcome or benefit . . . a lot of people have been concerned about developmental disabilities, retardation, deformities, things like that . . . that's one of the biggest concerns with eating mushrooms during pregnancy, breastfeeding, and the postpartum period." She noted, however, that if anything, the children were physically healthier, linguistically and otherwise ahead of their developmental markers.

[5]

Health Conditions Positively Affected

When I first heard about microdosing, I was very interested in what people were saying, but I found it hard to believe that one substance or even family of substances could do so many things.
—David Nutt[1]

Introduction

We are at the beginning of understanding how psychedelics work, and how microdosing works differently. We are further along in understanding how microdosing affects whole families of conditions because individuals testing microdoses on themselves have shared their experiences so generously.

At first, before this chapter came together, we might have agreed with Dr. Nutt. But as we became more and more aware of the diversity of conditions we were reviewing, and looked in detail at the evidence gathered so far, our opinion changed.

Even though the list of "so many things" that bothered Dr. Nutt was much smaller than what we are now reporting, it's easy to see how looking at each health condition with a specialized eye might magnify distinctions and strengthen incredulity.

However, when we stepped back from the obvious diversity and looked for commonalities, what we were struck by—especially for the conditions with no cure—is that there were other ways to view these conditions that fit the data better and made more sense.

Our task became to lay out enough of what we found so that individuals with any of these conditions, disorders, illnesses, or diseases would find enough here to help them make their own decisions about microdosing.

In a world where medicine is becoming ever more specialized, here are some generalizations about microdosing to help clarify things:

- Without exception, every physical condition in this list has a mental component, and every mental condition, a physical aspect. (Seems obvious, once stated.) Each condition is described, and then illustrated with real-life examples so that others can see if these examples illuminate their own condition. As you look over these conditions, we urge you to notice that, in almost every case, the first effect reported by people microdosing is that **they feel better.** Sometimes individuals point to an immediate difference like fewer migraines, or less depression or pain. More often, they notice their condition takes up less of their awareness and interferes less with their lives. It begins to make sense therefore that microdoses of psychedelics are positively affecting the overall body-mind system.

- After years of treatment for chronic conditions, most people stabilize or continue to decline, with declines slowed by treatments and medications. Remarkably, for a number of those conditions (including those for which at this point we only know of a single case), after microdosing was started, there was an improved level of relief, lessening of symptoms, and a greater return of function.

- With a few exceptions in dose level and sometimes protocols, microdosing for each condition is far more similar than the conditions themselves. We know it is unlikely that the same intervention will work for everyone. However, we also know that if an intervention works for one person, it may very well work for others with the same condition, although perhaps more or less effectively.

- Coming out of a world of data-driven research, we have been astounded, time after time, when we realize how much information was contained even in brief descriptions and how full a picture we can get from a single report.

- Many readers with specific conditions will skip directly to that section. After you do that, we suggest you look at a number of related conditions to more deeply understand the range of microdosing effects that may occur for you as well. Take a look at the overview and basic information provided in the first two chapters when you can.

Anorexia: A Case Study

From time to time, we present a single case in some detail. Some of these highlight conditions not necessarily associated with microdosing, and so are of special interest. Almost all scientific discovery begins with a single case—a single observation—often one that was unanticipated, unlooked for, or even contrary to what was expected. This case checks off all the boxes. Anorexia, also called anorexia nervosa, is an eating disorder where people lose more weight than is considered healthy for their age and height. The exact causes of anorexia nervosa are not known.

A study by the National Association of Anorexia Nervosa and Associated Disorders reported that between 5 and 10 percent of anorexics die within ten years after contracting the disease; 18 to 20 percent of anorexics will be dead after twenty years; and only 30 to 40 percent ever fully recover. The mortality rate associated with anorexia nervosa is twelve times higher than the death rate of all causes of death for females fifteen to twenty-four years old. And 20 percent of people suffering from anorexia will prematurely die from complications related to their eating disorder, including suicide and heart problems.[2]

In August 2023, we received an email from "K.M." "A thank you note" was its title.

> "I've been anorexic my whole life. I'm 40.
> I'm three months into my microdose journey.
> I've gained 30 lbs. My physical health has never been better, and my mental health has remained stable for so many consecutive weeks. I haven't induced vomiting for three weeks, reduced from 10–20 times a day. I'm considering returning to work after a twelve-year absence. I feel very privileged and pleased to be alive.
> Respect, from a grateful stranger."

Writing her back, Jim thanked her and asked if she could share in more detail. K.M. wrote back:

> "I only wish I'd journaled my story, but the truth is, I didn't believe it would work. I thought it would feel like every other anti-psychotic and psychiatric drug I've taken over the dismal years, but this isn't a drug. It's allowed me to access all the tools I've learned through therapy and never been able to engage."

She also enclosed a recent blog entry (edited for brevity and clarity):

> "My name is K., and I am an addict. That truth is my biggest shame, but this story is my proudest achievement.
> My addictions are varied . . . I lost 100 lbs. In Mexico I tried to become a crystal meth addict, because I thought it

might be an adventurous and skinny way to suicide. Yet I remained very much alive . . . I've been addicted . . . relentlessly and fruitlessly, I've been addicted to food, vomiting, starvation, and self-sabotage. A lifetime of self-flagellation . . .

Microdosing; I decided to microdose ketamine back when I lived in Goa, because I'd read about how it was changing lives, and healing minds. I bought a year's supply of ketamine and did it in two days and went missing for three weeks . . . I woke up from a coma in a Bangkok hospital.

My microdosing journey began three months ago. . . . Here I am in all my full-hipped, loud-mouthed glory. I've gained 30 lbs, I don't induce sickness from one week to the next. . . .

I will share this: a really important difference between an antidepressant and a psilocybin microdose. The function of an antidepressant is to turn off your sad. An antidepressant won't make you happy, but for some people it can extinguish some pain. A psilocybin microdose on the other hand, will actually increase happiness. It elevates one's mood in a way that no psychiatric drugs do. And, dear friends, it does that with no side effects whatsoever.

The best part is, I dose less each week than I did the week before. This isn't just a reasonable excuse for a new addiction. This is, thus far, by far the most beneficial psychiatric medication I've ever encountered.

I've spent the last three years trying to recover, but every time I reach the point of wellness, I become so afraid of life . . . of what addiction I'm going to replace starvation with, so that inevitably, I revert back to anorexia.

Microdosing has removed the fear. It's that simple. I am no longer afraid of the unknown. I want to live. I feel joy, and I want to feel it more. . . .

Identity: I have this toolbox filled with ways to self-soothe, ways to sit with emotion. Meditation, yoga, breathing exercises. I know all of those things can help me . . . but when I'm in a heightened emotional state, I found it impossible to access those skills. Since I've been microdosing psilocybin that changed. I can utilize those tools whenever I require them.

When I started microdosing, I used psilocybin to replace the urge to binge or purge whenever it arose. The first week I dosed .1g–.3g maybe two or three times a day. I was very aware that I was replacing one addiction with another, but this fresh one was pretty joyful, and I felt good, so I went with it.

I haven't had a dose for six days now.

I haven't consciously tried to limit my psilocybin use, I've just only used it when I've wanted to, and it happens that my wanting to microdose decreases as my vim for life increases."

It is important to recognize that her remarkable recovery owes much to her personal understanding, gained through years of suffering and therapy. By sufficiently reducing her anxiety, microdosing enabled her to make use of her hard-won understanding to take on a complex and serious condition.

It may well be that microdosing can become part of therapeutic protocols as a valuable, safe, and cost-effective treatment tool for anorexia and related conditions. In this case, it made a critical difference.

Anxiety

I've heard that microdosing might help anxiety, but others say to stay away from psychedelics entirely if this is what you're dealing with. What's right?

With certain conditions, our information changes over time.

During our early studies, the recommendation on the Microdosing Psychelics.com website was that microdosing for anxiety was contraindicated. Nevertheless, we received reports stating that people found that even generalized anxiety was relieved.

With many more years of reports, we can now be more specific. Anxiety appears to come in four general forms:

- Anxiety linked with other mental conditions, most commonly depression.
- Anxiety about something: a negative medical diagnosis, the behavior or condition of one's children, the security of one's job, and so on.
- Social anxiety in new situations and when interacting with new people, and in public speaking, resulting in withdrawal instead of contact.
- Undifferentiated, diffuse, or generalized anxiety: an overall feeling state that has no subject or focus.

Microdosing often benefits those suffering from the first three categories, with uneven results for generalized anxiety.

Anxiety linked with depression is often realistic: one's life is not working well—in part due to the depression. Close to 80 percent of the people who microdose for depression in our studies report considerable or total improvement. Their anxiety was reduced as well.

For people who have anxiety about a given situation, microdosing often improves the ability to resolve, cope with, or accept the situation. Anxiety is reduced accordingly.

The same seems true for the lessening of social anxiety across a wide range of conditions and reports.

For people with generalized anxiety, the results are mixed. Some individuals found microdosing increased the level of anxiety or their awareness of their anxiety while others found relief. We don't yet know why some people were successful and others were not. In any case, if microdosing raises your anxiety, first cut your dose in half. If unwanted effects persist, stop microdosing.

You can also get advice and support from a coach or therapist and determine, for example, if there are microdosing substance alternatives, like *Amanita muscaria,* or other helpful therapeutic modalities. *Amanita muscaria* shows particular promise online and off. As one article put it, "a huge catalog of anecdotal accounts states that the mushroom may ease anxiety and promote relaxation."[3]

Asthma Relief

If psychedelics are anti-inflammatories, will microdosing help my asthma?

An inflammatory disorder with multiple causes, asthma "is a condition in which airways narrow and swell making breathing difficult. For some people, it's a minor nuisance, but for others it can interfere with daily activities and even lead to a life-threatening asthma attack. Across the globe there are approximately 262 million people suffering from asthma, with that figure expected to rise over the next several decades."[4] Another source says, "its prevalence increases by 50% every decade."[5]

Allergic asthma is most common where "exposure to inhaled irritants, or triggers, can cause the walls of airways to become inflamed and the muscles around the airways to tighten up. That makes the airways narrower, leaving less room for air to flow."[6] Natural anti-inflammatories for treating asthma include green tea and omega-3 oils. While there are also many pharmaceutical medications—sometimes deployed through inhalers—these can cause tissue damage and a variety of other problems if used extensively over time.[7]

Real-world and laboratory evidence that microdosing can help those with asthma partly explains the ongoing scientific and commercial interest in the anti-inflammatory properties of psychedelics (further discussed in chapter 6). A 2020 study states: "Research has shown that psychedelics, such as lysergic acid diethylamide (LSD), have profound anti-inflammatory properties mediated by 5-HT(2A) receptor signaling, supporting their evaluation as a therapeutic for neuroinflammation associated with neurodegenerative disease."[8]

Real-World Reports

From Reddit

- "I started trials with microdosing. I am at about 0.1-gram shrooms and dose every 3rd day. I noticed to my amazement that the debilitating asthma I have had for the past 2 years, I am 59, is gone!"
- "I . . . have asthma and have also noticed that when I microdose it helps a lot with my breathing. It's like it opens up my lungs and feels wonderful."

From Our Files

"The asthma I have been experiencing came on suddenly after breathing cedar sawdust. Since then, I have not been able to raise my heart rate very much without my lungs closing down. It has been debilitating especially if I forget my puffer while hiking. Cold air, cold drink, dust, smoke from candles even, exertion all close down my lungs usually.

Well, even after two days from when I microdosed . . . I have spent the day burning brush, I brought my inhaler fully expecting to have to use it, and I didn't. I even ran up the hill to the house several times, a good heart pounding moderate sprint . . . no asthmatic response. Pretty strenuous activity making fire breaks too, and with sometimes unavoidable smoke . . . even a fraction of which would have shut down my lungs before . . . [now] nothing!

I have been using a nebulizer with glutathione which has been very helpful and stopped using it just to see. . . . My lungs have no symptoms. This is way more potent than any anti-inflammatory supplement . . . seems more on the level of steroids without side effects!"

Data from Baba Masha's 2022 book, *Microdosing with Amanita Muscaria—Creativity, Healing, and Recovery with the Sacred Mushroom,* suggests the potential efficacy of microdosing *Amanita muscaria.* Fourteen people in her asthma sample had "positive changes," while there were "No results" for twelve.[9]

This book is biased throughout toward paying attention more to individual reports than to restricted clinical studies, and rarely mentions work done only with animals (almost always laboratory mice or rats).

We feel that in this case, our preference for real-world experience is justified. This may not be true for other conditions.

Autism (Asperger's/High-Functioning)

Can microdosing help here?

The following question came in:

"Not quite sure even how to ask this question, but I'm described as having or being "Asperger's."* Nothing is wrong, and I have no need to function any more effectively. I have the

---

*Until 2013, "Asperger's"—named for the first person who described it—was a set of characteristics. In 2013, the professionals who regularly change the names and definitions of mental conditions decided to reclassify it as a form of autism that was "high-functioning," but on the same continuum as those who had low-functioning autism. We usually stick with the older definition, which we think is less confusing. People now often describe themselves as "being on the spectrum."

typical advantages over—and sensory and social processing issues with—neurotypicals.[10] Can microdosing be of any value?"

We have one suggestion, and a terrific referral. But first, an apology.

We are answering this question in our "health conditions" chapter. However, it doesn't fit there. According to Tim Jewell, "Neither what was previously diagnosed as Asperger's nor autism is a medical condition that needs to be 'treated.' Those diagnosed with autism are considered 'neurodivergent,'"[11] which is not a health "condition," as nothing needs to be changed or fixed.

Notable differences usually include high intelligence (especially analytic), incredible capacity to stay focused, and excellent attention to detail and complex structures. People with these characteristics gravitate to jobs in tech and other areas demanding comprehension of complex systems. It has been suggested that many Silicon Valley CEOs could be classified as Asperger's. Along with high capacities comes heightened sensory awareness, so that normal levels of noise, crowding, heat, and cold can be extremely uncomfortable. Often, individuals have a blunted awareness of subtle social cues—from social and work-related communications to intimate relationships—resulting in difficulties in maintaining connections with other people. For example, these individuals often cannot recognize which emotion is in play based on body language or voice tone, and are thus unable to tell if a remark is meant to be friendly, sarcastic, hostile, or a joke.

Microdosing at the dose levels described and referred to throughout this book will have little to no effect on people with Asperger's.

We rarely can be this definite, but when Jim and Sophia Korb were collecting their first few hundred cases, a number of people reported that microdosing had no effect until they increased their LSD dose to at least fifty micrograms (normal range is seven to twelve). At that dose level, the effects were similar to what other people were reporting.

Neither Jim nor Sophia had any idea at the time why this was so. However, in 2017, Jim received an email: "My name is Aaron, and

I identify as a psychedelic advocate and psychedelic-therapist-to-be." He described himself as being on the autistic spectrum. They corresponded, and it soon became clear that Aaron had read almost everything relevant to becoming a psychedelic therapist, and had extensive personal knowledge of the effects of varying doses of psychedelics. He understood how psychedelics had not only benefited him, but how they could benefit others with his characteristics. As there were no training programs that met his needs, he continued his own research.

This led to the 2020 publication of Aaron Orsini's first book, *Autism on Acid: How LSD Helped Me Understand, Navigate, Alter & Appreciate My Autistic Perceptions*. It describes in detail the difficulties of growing up being unable to recognize social cues and assess others' emotional states. Imagine if, when anyone speaks to you, you don't know whether they have said it kindly, in anger, affectionately, or sarcastically. Every conversation entails endless inner analysis and guessing meanings that come unconsciously and automatically for neurotypicals.

Orsini has laid out high-functioning autism's inner world. He's been able to explain all this to neurotypicals thanks to his extensive experimentation with psychedelics, which helped him find ways to overcome the problems he'd faced. He was able to "clean the windows," so to speak, so that his natural intellectual advantages were not limited by a struggle to guess the meaning of normal social behavior. He became equally adept in both worlds.

This book led to other publications, a website, a Facebook page, and currently a thriving worldwide community devoted to people helping each other and improving on or overcoming what had previously been considered disadvantages. In addition to developing this support network, Orsini leads a Royal College of London research team doing formal research on the effects of psychedelics on those with Asperger's. While there are many organizations supporting those with Asperger's, the only one we know of focused on the proper use of low doses is Orsini's, at autisticpsychedelic.com.

Update: A report posted to the microdosing subreddit on Reddit is suggestive of the range of changes possible for individuals high on the spectrum:

> "I was diagnosed with autism. I'll have an insane tunnel vision that disables me from doing anything else other than what I'm focused on for an entire day. I would previously go 12 hours without eating and have anxiety all day before micro-dosing LSD. Now food actually tastes good, I smoke less weed because I look forward to actually eating. I am a lot better at multitasking. I feel like I can put my mind to anything I want to put my mind to, and not in a manic-depressive way. Overall, it's been a month of taking small doses . . . and I've noticed no ill side effects . . . no hallucinations. Even my vision is just brighter, it seemed as if I was seeing in black and white before and now there's life! I have 0 anxiety when I take LSD."

Autism (Severe) and Children

What about giving microdoses to a child diagnosed as being on the spectrum?

It's too early to say much about autism and children. However, there are some reports and even forgotten but important research.

At one point, Jim was asked by a parent with considerable personal psychedelic experience if it would be all right to give a microdose to a five-year-old child diagnosed with severe autism. His response:

> I told him it was not something I could recommend, as we knew little about the effects of psychedelics on very young children. Generally speaking, most medications, especially those that might affect brain functioning, are not recommended.

The father went ahead anyway, having determined what he considered an appropriate dose for his child. Several days later, he sent this message: "[My son] became much more social and used many more words than usual. He was happier, and he did not hit his head on the floor nearly as much as he normally does."

Three years later, an update: the father says his child, now eight, takes a low dose of LSD about once a month. "He is more and more capable of sustained interest in things. We spend a lot of time in nature together; we live near a creek, and he gets fascinated by it all. The LSD helps him reset emotionally. He becomes more calm, more focused, and enjoys himself more long after the dose."

Currently, according to government sources, in the US alone, millions of children with various kinds of learning difficulties are given daily doses of stimulants. Paradoxically, in many cases, these children become better able to focus in school, stop being disruptive, and report that they appreciate being able to regulate their feelings and behaviors themselves. Why mention this? To reinforce the need for caution when considering giving mind-altering substances to children. They are not simply tiny adults, and do not react as adults do.

As for microdosing and the autism spectrum disorder (ASD), the work done by psychedelic research pioneers Gary Fisher, Loretta Bender, and others with schizophrenic and autistic children has sadly been forgotten. Consider some of their results, as reported in *The Psychedelic Explorer's Guide* (Fadiman, 2011):

> In an analysis of the seven studies available, of 91 children
> ages 5 to 15 who were given a wide range of doses of LSD in
> a variety of settings, 75 of the children showed either good or
> excellent improvement.[12]

As we learned from a personal communication, one little girl (on more than a microdose) came over to psychologist Gary Fisher, who was sitting at one end of the room. She put her hand on his knee, looked up at him, and said, "We're all one, aren't we?" Dr. Fisher nodded in agreement. The little girl turned back and went to be with the other children. Prior to this, she had not spoken in several years. As psychedelic research was curtailed by law soon after this event, the study was never followed up on, and to this date has not been repeated.

Binge Eating

When I googled "microdosing and binge eating," several articles said high doses of MDMA and psychedelics might be helpful. Do you know anything more?

We do have a few encouraging reports. Binge eating is a psychological condition where a person feels out of control. On the one hand, they are overeating foods that normally give them pleasure, but at the same time, because they overeat to obvious excess, they're usually left physically uncomfortable, and ashamed or guilty for their lack of control. It's almost always with comfort food—nobody ever binges on brussels sprouts—but goes way past the point of being comforting.

According to the National Institutes of Health, binge eating "is the most common eating disorder in the U.S."[13] The Mayo Clinic says that the causes of binge eating are unknown, but then adds that "genetic, biological factors, long term dieting, and psychological issues increase your risk." If you reread that, it sounds like a longer and classier way of saying, "the causes are unknown." While it's a little scary to take issue with anything the Mayo Clinic says, they do seem to classify binge eating as if it were a disease, when it seems more likely that it's a coping mechanism, and in that sense is more cultural and psychological.

If someone is binge eating to feel better, from a whole person perspective, it's not that different from other activities and behaviors we do to feel better that also don't work in excess, such as social drinking, tobacco and cannabis smoking, and even exercise. This would then also include porn, computer games, and to a lesser extent, social media.

In our reports from those who have microdosed for binge eating, what's most striking is that they did not seem to try to consciously increase their intention, or double down on their willpower, or use any of the psychological practices suggested in the literature and self-help materials on binge eating. Instead, it is as if their mind-body system rebalanced itself, and their excessive behavior simply stopped. Here are excerpts from those reports:

- "I struggle with binge eating disorder and now it is 2 weeks after I started microdosing 100mg every other day and I have not binged yet! I usually binge 5 days a week lol, is there any research on this? I feel like I have control over myself now."
- "I'm not a binge eater but I drink a lot of soda. I have been drinking water since I started, and I've had a box of my favorite cookies sitting on the shelf for a week unopened. It's really weird to me, but I'm ok with it."
- "I've never really thought about it before, but I've been better at snacking less. Or at least snacking better and not eating half a jar of peanut butter every night. 😄"

Bipolar Disorder

Any research or report on those diagnosed with or self-reporting as bipolar being helped? Is it safe to microdose if I or someone in my family has a bipolar diagnosis?

A common definition of bipolar disorder is "a mental health condition that causes a wide range of mood episodes, from low-energy moods to high-energy moods."[14] It used to be called "manic-depressive" disorder, which was considerably more descriptive. It is genetically linked.

If a woman has the condition, there is a 10 percent chance that it will be passed on to her children. It is considered to be a lifelong condition.

According to the National Institute of Mental Health, "An effective treatment plan usually includes a combination of medication and psychotherapy, also called talk therapy."[15] Bipolar affects approximately eight million adults in the US and approximately forty million individuals worldwide.[16]

Microdosing often alleviates depression, releasing bound energy to make possible other life improvements.[17] The idea that microdosing might be helpful for those diagnosed or self-reporting as bipolar is regularly discussed on Reddit.

However, there is no *published* evidence about safety or lack of safety with higher doses. This is because almost every published clinical study of high-dose psychedelics excludes individuals with psychotic or bipolar episodes in their past and usually eliminates anyone with a family history of such episodes.

A few years ago, Jim wrote to one well-known researcher and asked if there was any evidence that high doses of psychedelics had *actually* caused such episodes. He received back a number of papers, some by other researcher friends. All repeated the exclusion—almost by rote. None of the studies reported that an episode had ever occurred. The assumption is still widely shared in the therapeutic community.

Jim then found a bipolar support group page on Facebook. He asked the moderator if he could ask group members if they'd had any psychedelic experience, one way or another. The general advice of these support group members was that high-dose psychedelics could be very beneficial *if taken during the depressed part of a bipolar cycle,* but they felt—and a number had experienced—that taking a high-dose psychedelic during a manic episode or even a milder hypomanic episode was like pouring gasoline on a fire. Not recommended. As this was a while ago, no one mentioned microdosing. And no one said that their psychedelic sessions had changed their diagnosis.

The best answer we can give right now is that if someone with a personal or family background of bipolar disorder wishes to microdose, they should begin during a depressed part of their cycle and have access to a microdosing professional, coach, or an informed good friend, in case support is needed. It's especially important to start with a low dose.

It makes us a little bit nervous to go against the well-established protocols that prevent people with bipolar diagnosis from participating in high-dose research, but as microdoses do not trigger the intense reactions that concern high-dose researchers, used appropriately, microdosing is likely to be safe and may very well be therapeutic.

Body Weight

Will microdosing help me lose (or gain) weight?

After reviewing two recent reports from individuals who felt that microdosing played a critical role in their weight loss (of 70 and 130 pounds, respectively), there are clearly cases where *microdosing helps maintain focus and attention, supports healthier habit patterns, and can facilitate a shift in food preferences.*

Microdosing, by itself, will not necessarily lead to weight loss. Sorry, there's no magic bullet here. On the other hand, it likely does make it easier. So while it lacks the obscurity, mystique, and price of the many magic diet pills you will find on the internet, we do have many reports of people shifting their eating patterns toward a better and healthier weight, even when that's not what they were microdosing for.

The body strives for health, just as the mind strives for sanity and clarity. Microdosing supports these strivings, and because of that should be considered as an adjunct to any seriously intended weight loss (or weight gain) program that represents a return to a healthier equilibrium.

Cannabis Reduction or Quitting

Can microdosing help here?

The following inquiry came in:

> "Can microdosing really help me quit weed? I've quit weed
> multiple times. . . . One time I stopped for about three weeks
> and was so depressed I started again. . . . I recently started mi-
> crodosing, hoping it will get me through the depressing part.
> Please, if you have any positive stories, I'd love to hear them."

Cannabis (marijuana) is a safe pleasure for most people, and for
many, therapeutic. It can, however, become a vitality-draining depen-
dency. It is becoming increasingly clear that overuse brings real health
risks. There is increasing evidence that "cannabis is associated with serious heart complications—including heart attack and stroke."[18] Also,
more cannabis is being bred to have very high THC levels (at the cost
of decreasing CBD and other beneficial compounds), which can lead to
"cannabis use disorder" (which looks like addiction) or even psychosis.[19]

Quitting (or even cutting back) is not easy for some people, and
there's no one-size-fits-all way to go about it. A variety of reports show
how some people who struggled with cannabis were successful with
the help of microdosing in reducing their use or eventually stopping
completely.

- "I quit in 2005 and it was the best thing I ever did. . . . Then,
  I started up again last year. It was the worst thing I ever did. I
  miss who I was. But [with microdosing] I'm getting me back,
  little by little. . . . I can feel real joy and contentment and be
  more present in the moment without it. I'm more productive
  and present with my family, following through with my re-
  sponsibilities and goals."

- "Been a daily evening smoker for 6 years and could never quit. Since I started microdosing last month, I just don't want it. The shrooms make it so much easier to recognize why I craved weed, so I can better push aside the urges."

- "I've taken breaks from weed here and there but was never able to fully quit until micro and macro dosing! . . . I have clear thoughts, sharper focus, way less grogginess. I feel much lighter without weed in my life."

- "It works. When I MD I can go all day in a flow state and not even realize I haven't smoked, LOL. MD is amazing for this when used properly."

- "Three weeks today with nothing at all!"

- "It took me a couple months for the craving and habitual misuse to fade into the background . . . for me, it was causing anxiety/depression. . . . Microdosing helped me realize this and make the connection. . . . I haven't smoked weed in 9 months, and I couldn't be happier."

- "Saving about $600 a month! Had been a daily smoker for 30 years."

- "It's helped me reduce my desire for daily tokes. Before, I would notice the irritability of withdrawal during the day and have a puff here or there, thinking I was irritated by life not weed withdrawal. LOL. Microdosing has made that irritability and desire much less, though not eliminated it."

In short, for some people, microdosing made it easier to cut down or quit entirely.

Cerebral Palsy: A Case Study

Cerebral palsy (CP) is a group of disorders that affect a person's ability to move and maintain balance and posture. It is caused by abnormal development of the brain, or damage to the developing brain before birth, that affects a person's ability to control their muscles.

There is no cure for CP, but treatment can improve the lives of those who have the condition. And it is "non-progressive," that is, it does not get worse with age.[20]

We have a single case.

Birgitta is a thirty-three-year-old Dutch woman who recently completed her PhD. She was diagnosed with cerebral palsy a few months after her birth. She does not use medication and attributes her good physical condition in part to early physiotherapy.

She describes herself as healthy, and not in any pain except when she pulls a muscle, "something that everybody has every few months." She continues with physical therapy to prevent a slight curvature of her spine from getting any worse.

For the past six months, she has been microdosing under the guidance of a coach and has been given an unusual protocol: alternating LSD (five micrograms) every fourth day with mushrooms (0.2 grams) plus lion's mane and Syrian rue. Her coach explains:

> "Why I've decided to have Birgitta on both is mostly intuitive and my understanding of each medicine. . . . LSD as an agent of empowerment . . . carries the potential to rewire and lay down new neural networks. . . . I have my own personal bias with LSD as I'm in awe of its potential.
>
> Psilocybin works somatically, like a conductor tuning up an out-of-tune orchestra."

Birgitta herself also describes her experiences (edited for brevity and clarity):

> "When I started taking the medicines, I immediately noticed a much greater appreciation of nature. This was something I

was already working on . . . I think the mushrooms acceler-
ated the process. Particularly at the start, I would sit in the
garden and feel in the presence of the trees and other plants
as if they were conscious entities, particularly on mushroom
days. Throughout this time, I have had a slight difficulty dropping off to sleep on mushroom days and sometimes I have to
use a bit of CBD to relax.

I feel a much greater effect on LSD days than on mushroom days. LSD intensifies whatever I am working on.

If I want to work, I am really focused and get a lot done.

If I want to interact with another person, I feel really
connected to them.

If I am reading something, I get really into what I am reading and forget to stop.

I also feel calm and able to observe and analyze my emotions on LSD.

My parents don't know about my medicine use because
they would just see it as drug misuse and blame my assistants
in some way. Even with a doctorate, my parents don't think I
should deviate from their way of thinking.

Last week, I was talking to my father about my career. He
said, in the last six or seven months, I have moved from needing his guidance in the world of work to being on an equal
level with him. This corresponds exactly to the time I have
been with the medicine.

My mother and my assistants have told me that they find
my movement disorder to be less pronounced in the last few
months.

In terms of mood, I have already always been an extremely
positive person. However, people around me [now] are always
hearing me say that I am living in the happiest time of my
life."

Cluster Headaches

Can microdosing stop them or lower their painfulness?

There is considerable evidence that high doses of psychedelics help cluster headache sufferers. More recently, small doses as well as larger doses have been found effective. The current consensus on how psychedelics can halt or lessen cluster headaches provides a model of effective citizen science.

Basic information: Cluster headaches, different from and far more debilitating than migraines, are among the most painful conditions experienced by human beings. They are often called "suicide headaches," as sufferers commit suicide at a rate twenty-two times that of the general population. A bout of clusters may continue for several weeks to several months, each episode lasting one to three hours. The frequency of occurrence ranges from every other day to multiple times a day. The cause of cluster headaches is unknown, and it often takes years to even get a correct diagnosis.

The best and most current information comes from Clusterbusters .org, a nonprofit established to advocate for research and funding on cluster headaches and to disseminate information on the effective use of psychedelics in pain relief.

Clusterbusters' protocols are based on years of relieving people's previously intractable pain. Originally, Clusterbusters advocated high doses. Most recently, they have revised their protocols, which focus both on dealing with cluster cycles once they have started, as well as preventing cycles from starting in the first place. They now recommend low doses to start, close to the dose range for microdosing.[21] A typical dose might be 1.5 grams, which the afflicted individual will undertake once every five days—a unique protocol called the "pulse regimen"—to attempt to interrupt the cycle of coming cluster headaches.[22]

Nothing that we know of completely cures cluster headaches. However, many individuals have effectively controlled their cluster headaches with small doses. As Clusterbusters puts it, "Many cluster headache sufferers . . . find that small, sub-hallucinogenic doses of these tryptamines can end cluster headache cycles and prevent entire cycles from starting."[23]

The full story of how Clusterbusters began and created a novel citizen science research program is the core of the book *Psychedelic Outlaws: The Movement Revolutionizing Modern Medicine* (Kempner, 2024).

Takeaway: Psychedelics at different dose levels have been more successful than any other intervention. If you suffer from cluster headaches, go to their site for more information.

Color Blindness (Red-Green)

Is color blindness a contraindicated condition? Being red-green color blind, I was told I shouldn't microdose. Is that right?

The answer is a bit complicated. When Jim and Sophia originally collected information about microdosing's effects on all kinds of conditions, several people reported that after a microdose—and for several days after—they would see tracers* (streaks or trails of light) coming from bright lights, ceiling lights, reading lights, and so on. They finally figured out that each of those individuals had red-green color deficiency (someone who lacks the cells to perceive green or red or both). They also found that lots of people see tracers after taking high doses.

Sophia came up with a real-world evidence test. She asked a friend with strong red-green color blindness if he would microdose. When he did, he saw tracers for the next two days.

We added a warning to our microdosingpsychedelics.com informa-

---

*Technically, *palinopsia* is the persistence or recurrence of a visual image after the stimulus has been removed. It looks like the after-tail of a sparkler being moved in the dark.

tional website: those with red-green color blindness should not microdose as they would likely experience tracers after each dose. Since very few people have the condition, that's where things have stayed.

However, telling people who want to try a new way to take psychedelics that they can't is like handing a bean to a six-year-old child and saying, "Don't put this bean up your nose."

As microdosing became more and more popular, more people with red-green color deficiency saw the warning. Some went ahead anyway, and some of them had tracers. However, their reports generally stated that the advantages of microdosing outweighed their discomfort. In every other way, their results were in the normal range.

If you have red-green color deficiency, it's your decision.

Common Cold

Can microdosing help me to get over my cold?

It might very well, but we have little specific information. There has been no research for this condition, and we have only one written report.

While the common cold may seem of minimal concern, a multibillion-dollar industry exists solely to reduce the suffering and minimize the duration of people's discomfort. As for whether microdoses can help achieve these goals, Jim received this email note from an anthropologist:

> "Whenever I feel the beginnings of a cold,
> I take a bite from a dried mushroom.
> For the last 20 years,
> I have not had a single cold."

While it is tempting to speculate as to whether this may be more generally true, you now know as much as we do. Make your own experiments, come to your own conclusions, and let us know what you find out by contacting us through the MicrodosingBook.com website.*

Dizziness (Perpetual): A Case Study

"My husband had continual dizziness (PPPD). He has tried all the therapies prescribed over the last few months with little improvement. Microdosing was different."

Persistent postural perceptual dizziness—PPPD—has three main symptoms: dizziness, vertigo, and swaying. PPPD symptoms may come and go throughout the day, with episodes lasting up to several hours. And on most days they occur for an indefinite period of time. In a 2021 study of 198 individuals with PPPD, people experienced symptoms for a median duration of 1.5 years and an average duration of 3.5 years.[24] "In PPPD, the normal 'filters' that the brain uses to suppress feelings of movement that we need not be conscious of, go wrong. Instead of the brain being able to balance everything up and give you a nice smooth feeling when you are moving, the person can feel a sense of movement that they shouldn't."[25]

Jim corresponded with a woman whose husband was dizzy all the time. Nothing ordinary science or medicine saw or measured explained why it was happening or what could be done about it. He took every treatment offered for PPPD, including antidepressants (because he felt terrible).

When he first microdosed, he felt better emotionally. After he'd been microdosing for several weeks, he felt better than he had for years and could be social without taking a rest afterward. His whole situation had positively shifted, including considerable improvement with the PPPD itself.

As he'd tried *everything* else he'd been recommended—and nothing had helped—from his perspective, whatever was offered next wasn't

---

*Elsewhere in the book we are dismissive of a single dose. Here, however, we give it its due.

likely to be any different. When he was approached with microdosing, he said he didn't have the "faintest idea" whether it might help. For him, it was just treatment number twelve in a long line of unsuccessful treatments. He had no reason to think this would be any different.

And yet it worked. Perhaps in this and similar cases, microdosing is helpful even without a placebo boost.

Eczema

I've had eczema since I was a kid. It gets better, it gets worse; treatment helps, treatment doesn't help. Any idea if microdosing can get me off this merry-go-round?

As is true with many conditions, current medical science suggests there are many causes of eczema, and offers many symptomatic treatments, but offers no more than that. Here is what the National Eczema Association says about the condition:

> Eczema is the name for a group of inflammatory skin conditions that cause itchiness, dry skin, rashes, scaly patches, blisters and skin infections. . . . More than 31 million Americans have some form of eczema. Eczema can begin during childhood, adolescence, or adulthood—and it can range from mild to severe.
>
> Newborn babies can experience eczema within the first few weeks and months after birth. Young children with eczema can experience patches of skin that are extremely dry; itchy skin that can lead to blisters and skin infections due to excessive scratching. Adults can also experience eczema and adult eczema is most commonly developed when someone is in their 20s or over the age of 50. . . .
>
> Atopic dermatitis, the most common type of eczema . . . results from an overactive immune system that causes the skin

barrier to become dry and itchy. This condition can occur on any part of the body and has varied symptoms.[26]

This encouraging report was sent to the microdose coach Adam Bramlage, who shared it with us:

"I've been dealing with chronic eczema for the past 20 years. I've had to deal with itchy red rashes on my hands, arms and legs, cracked knuckles that bleed and limit my dexterity, also sores that express moisture and yellow pus. Needless to say, it's been a very uncomfortable journey.

Before I started my [microdosing] regimen, I experienced one of the worst outbreaks I'd ever had.

As soon as I began microdosing, I noticed very significant improvements within a day, cracks closing up faster, better mobility, and then ongoing progress both physically and mentally with the eczema receding and my overall attitude being lifted. I continue to take them [microdoses] and I'm still seeing improvements."

As is true with the other single cases reported here, we hope this one will encourage those with this condition to consider microdosing. Our second reason for including single cases is to draw researchers' attention to microdosing's effects on these conditions to evaluate whether more formal research may be appropriate. We like to read the phrase "No Cure" optimistically, as "No Cure Yet."

Ehlers-Danlos Syndrome and an Accident: A Case Study

Rose has Ehlers-Danlos syndrome (EDS), a genetic disorder that affects her body's ability to produce the collagen necessary to support her body's connective tissues. The primary symptoms are hypermobility, joint instability, and chronic pain. Instability means that the joints don't hold together well. A simple quick movement of one's head, for example, can result in a dislocation that needs treatment for months. More severe injuries are common.

Although there is currently no cure for EDS, a varity of treatments exist for specific symptoms.

Now aged sixty, Rose displayed hypermobility from early childhood. "When I was four or five, I could sit in any position—bottoms of my feet touching, knees at an angle touching the floor, or like a frog with legs behind me with knees on each side to the ground, and sit in any yoga position." She experienced no negative effects until after the birth of her child at age thirty-seven. Since that time, she has had three operations for joint replacement, with constant pain as an aftereffect.

Twenty years ago, she had a serious accident. "I have been in chronic disabling pain for over twenty years daily since I broke my back falling down a flight of stairs with my infant in my arms, landing on the center of my spine cradling the baby." It was necessary to fuse parts of her back so she could function. She began to take pain medications, some of which had serious negative effects but were necessary to keep her pain at a bearable level so she could raise her two children and continue her business career.

Rose's Microdosing History

"September 16, 2022

My first dose was a capsule with 150 milligrams of psilocybin, 150 milligrams of lion's mane, and 100 milligrams of niacin that I bought in an open-air farmers market in a small town in Mexico.

Microdosing: every other day for the 1st 2 doses. Felt like too much on my brain. Sort of seasick and heavy (but sleep was great and pain subsided overnight). Now every 3rd day to present.

October 22, 2022

Waking up is different now. Before microdosing, someone would have to rouse me from sleep, and I would have to laboriously push through webs of myofascial, nerve, and muscle pain to even form words. I would take lethal doses of ibuprofen, an opioid, and depression and anxiety meds while lying flat. It would take 20–40 minutes after taking the meds before I could sit up without searing pain (but still with substantial pain), let alone walk. With my first stand and step, my energy for the day would begin to just pour from my body. A shower or interaction early guaranteed exhaustion for the day.

Weather would exacerbate this. Rain, cold, seasonal changes, humidity, barometric changes, etcetera. Today, it is cold, raining cats and dogs, and the room I woke in is chilly.

I woke up on my own and without moving, looked around with my eyes, curious what the day would bring. I gently realized, I felt no nerve, muscle, or myofascial pain. I felt like a child. It reminded me of that moment when I'd wake up before my mom and smile, knowing I could find something fun to do myself before anyone else woke.

I didn't feel like a senior in my body. I felt like I did as a kid. Even my mind felt the joy, wondering what a new day would bring, not "How am I going to get through today?"

Microdosing has improved my sleep . . . I wake rested and pain-free. My fibromyalgia, and rheumatoid and osteoarthritis pain, have subsided to such a low level I'm only vaguely aware they exist. My major joint pain is still present, but the inflammation surrounding these areas is gone, making it much easier to move. My fingers were so swollen from arthritis inflammation and so disfigured, I could not move them freely. Now I can, and the swelling is down. My hand pain always woke me at night, as did my toe pain; both are calm and do not wake me.

Medications Before and Now

Substance	Before	Now
Duloxetine	60 mg 1/day	60 mg 1/day
Wellbutrin-Bupropion	150 mg 1/day	Tapered off. None.
Hydrocodone	5–325 2–3/day	1/day for major joint pain or total joint replacements in back, hip, and knees
Ibuprofen	800 mg 2/day	None
Omeprazole	Daily for acid reflux	Pepcid—as needed
Lyrica, taken for 20 years for pain	75 mg, 1–2, 3/day and 3–4 OK at night (never took that much)	None
Soma, taken for 20 years for pain	350 mg 2–3/day	None

I walked and moved like the Tin Man for decades. Today I feel like the Scarecrow! I can dance! I never thought I would dance again.

Smoking: I smoked socially in my teens and 20s. I smoked on and off until I discovered I was pregnant. That day I quit cold turkey. Decades later, I would still crave cigarettes. Since microdosing, the cravings for cigarettes have gone away entirely. What a relief.

Drinking: I loved drinking as a young adult and socially drank without even thinking much about it throughout life. Now, I am also uninterested in alcohol—completely.

Neither was a goal I had in mind before or mostly while microdosing.

Summary: The quality of my life is beyond anything it's been since I busted my back. I am able to listen, hear, and share myself without the layer of pain defense so active before that it blocked me from truly being present with the ones I love.

My oldest son, upon seeing me now, remarked, 'Wow! You are right here! Present. There is nothing between us for the first time in my life!'

My damaged and replaced joints still hurt, don't get me wrong. I have a lifetime of worn-out parts. But the pain is isolated to its part, manageable, and lets me know where there is still actual damage or injury. I do take a daily hydrocodone for my joint pain directly and occasionally get steroid injections for my joints, deteriorating due to EDS hypermobility. The difference is that now my body and mind aren't overwhelmed."

Epilepsy

Can microdosing help with this condition?

Epilepsy is a condition in which nerve cell activity in the brain is disturbed, causing seizures. It may result from a genetic disorder or an acquired brain injury, such as a trauma or stroke. (Seizures occur for many other reasons, including some medications.) Symptoms are treated with medication, and in more severe cases, with diet therapy, nerve stimulation, or surgery. To date, it cannot be cured.

It is generally thought that psychedelics are *not* a wise choice for epileptics: "There is a paucity of scientific information to support [psilocybin's] efficacy as a psychotherapy agent for epileptics. As a result, playing it safe and using recommended medication is much more advisable."[27] We did not find reports of epileptics using psychedelics successfully with LSD or LSD microdosing.

However, there is evidence of positive microdosing results for epilepsy with *Amanita muscaria*. Masha states that while her data, based on the reports of native Russians, is limited, "Positive results were noted by 77% (17 of 22) of participants; no effect, 14% (3) of cases, and negative effects . . . in 9% (2)."[28]

There is also *considerable evidence of CBD's effectiveness*. While that's outside this book's scope, we've included some important and hopefully helpful articles in this endnote.[29]

Headaches (Migraine)

Is it true that microdosing is effective at reducing migraines?

There is evidence that even a single large dose of psilocybin can substantially benefit migraine sufferers. As a published 2020 study called "Exploratory Controlled Study of the Migraine-Suppressing Effects of Psilocybin" found, "there is an enduring therapeutic effect in migraine headache after a single administration of psilocybin. The separation of acute psychotropic effects and lasting therapeutic effect is an important finding."[30]

Our concern here is focused on microdoses for migraine sufferers. Very early on, when Jim first realized that microdosing might affect physical symptoms as well as mental ones, he received two reports, both from the wives of holistic physicians who'd had chronic migraine headaches over many years. The women's reports were joyful little notes, each saying that they'd gone a good week, ten days, or as long as they could remember going without a migraine. Jim had hoped that with microdosing, they might have become migraine-free.

He wrote one of the women to ask how she was doing. She replied, "Last week I had a migraine that lasted 36 hours." Jim wrote back saying he was sad for her pain and sorry that it had happened. Her reply was unexpected:

> "I don't think you quite understand what's happened for me. That was *one* headache—in a month!! I used to have them for 20 days or more—every month."

Each of these women reported independently that, while the frequency and intensity of her migraines had diminished considerably, they were not gone completely.

Both of these women had previously tried—without success—mainstream medical solutions and herbal, homeopathic, and other treatments.

Later, after collecting hundreds of individual reports about migraines, a similar pattern emerged. Most people did report great relief, but almost no one reported complete remission. When people now ask whether microdosing will help with migraine headaches, the answer becomes, "Yes, it's highly likely it will help, but equally likely you will still have them now and then."

Inflammatory Bowel Disease (IBD)

How could microdosing help my Crohn's?

Crohn's disease is one of a family of closely related inflammatory bowel diseases (along with ulcerative colitis) that make up inflammatory bowel disease (IBD). It can cause inflammation in any part of the digestive tract. Symptoms include abdominal pain, severe diarrhea, fatigue, weight loss, and malnutrition. It is considered a progressive disease—it gets worse over time—and its causes are considered both genetic and environmental. While dietary changes are often suggested, most sources agree with the Mayo Clinic that "IBD treatment usually involves either drug therapy or surgery."[31]

Having received reports that microdosing seemed to help, we spoke with Andrew Kornfield, the former CEO of IBD Coach, a company that helps IBD patients reduce inflammation and related symptoms through guided lifestyle changes that diminish or eliminate drug use and help prevent surgery.

According to Andrew:

Psychedelics directly and indirectly modulate the immune system, alter the microbiome, and foster neuroplasticity. Together, these mechanisms influence the Microbiome-Gut-Brain Axis ("MGB axis"). Microdosing appears to provide patients with similar benefits in a more consistent manner, without the profound alterations in consciousness associated with full psychedelic experiences. In my personal work with hundreds of patients with IBD, dozens of people, microdosing and following dietary strategies and lifestyle changes, have reported mental benefits and notable reductions in symptoms. As part of working with conditions like IBD, microdosing appears to enhance adherence, foster acceptance, and amplify the efficacy of such approaches.[32]

As the science becomes more developed, the impact of microdosing on the MGB axis will likely be clarified.

For now, we have many reports like the following: "Not sure why, but changing my diet got easier (but still hard) after I added micro-dosing to my program. And was also able to cut back on some meds without pain." Given the large number of people who have reported positive diet shifts, it seems likely that part of what microdosing does is improve the functioning of the MGB axis.

Libido Lacking

If I've been low in the libido department for a while, could microdosing help?

Yes, maybe it can, and not because it's somehow equivalent to Viagra or some other magic "love drug" pharmaceutical but because of how microdosing enhances physical health as well as relationships. Please take a look at "Sexual Enhancement" in chapter 3.

Lupus: A Case Study

I have terrible lupus. I'm on many medications and get very little relief. My husband read that microdosing helps a lot of different things. Please answer.

Lupus is an autoimmune disease. The immune system of the body mistakenly attacks healthy tissue. It can affect the skin, joints, kidneys, brain, and other organs. Lupus has no cure. The only goal of treatment is to control symptoms.

After receiving this somewhat desperate request, Jim responded that it was unclear if microdosoing could help. The wife decided to order truffle microdoses from the Netherlands and said that she and her husband would both observe any changes in her symptoms and report back.

Although she had experienced the first symptoms of lupus after the birth of her daughter in 1992, it was not diagnosed until 2003.

The couple created a checklist of thirty symptoms, each to be ranked from zero to ten. Zero was nothing wrong, ten was severe. The symptoms included migraines, skin lesions, areas of pain, brain fog, rashes, sleep disturbances, reduced sex drive, and suicidal ideation. She recorded her daily symptoms for seven months.

During her first week of microdosing, there was a steep decline in symptoms. Over the months she kept records, her symptoms continued to decrease, briefly returning to higher levels when she was stressed.

Before she started, she was on fifteen medications. She was able to go off seven of them within a month. In 2024, she remained on eight medications and hormone replacement therapy for menopause.

Her lupus symptoms scores continued to decline numerically, but not enough for her to really feel the difference. She says things remain stable when she maintains her microdosing protocol.

Brief Summary of Results

Time Period	June 2021, first day of microdosing	January 2022, last week of daily recording	January 2024, one day only in response to follow-up request
Total Symptoms Score	Day 1, 215; by day 7, it had fallen to 116	Day 1, 49; day 7, 54	43
Number of Symptoms Scoring 4 or Higher	21	3 (fatigue, sleep, and reduced sex drive)	5 (stomach and indigestion, fatigue, reduced sex drive, and fibromyalgia pain)
Numbers of Symptoms Scoring 0	1 (migraine)	18	16

Lyme Disease
(Persistent Lyme Disease Syndrome)

Is there any evidence as to microdosing success with persistent or post-treatment Lyme disease?

While we don't know *how* it helps, we do have a few remarkable cases showing that it *can* help.

Background: "Lyme disease is caused by the bacterium Borrelia burgdorferi and rarely, Borrelia mayonii. It is transmitted to humans through the bite of infected blacklegged ticks. Typical symptoms include fever, headache, fatigue, and a characteristic skin rash called erythema migrans. Lyme disease is the most common vector-borne disease (that is, a disease transmitted by mosquitoes, ticks, or fleas) in the United States."[33]*

---

*Lyme specialists suggest that this is only a partial description. For alternative therapies and other bacteria that may be involved, see, e.g., Restorative Health Solutions at https://www.lymedr.com/home.

In recent years, approximately twenty to thirty thousand confirmed cases of Lyme disease per year have been reported to the Centers for Disease Control and Prevention. *Consumer Reports* estimates the number at more like half a million Americans each year, with serious symptoms including severe arthritis and irregular heart rhythms.[34] The number of cases reported in the United States has doubled in the last few years, and, while it's primarily found in the New England states, over 40 states have reported at least one infection. It's also found in most other parts of the world.

The tick bite transmits several different strains of bacteria, which in turn can cause a cascade of symptoms. In most cases, if treated early enough, it can be controlled with several weeks to months of continuous antibiotics.

It seem improbable that a system-wide condition caused by bacteria that is remarkably resistant to treatment would be affected by psychedelics, let alone by microdosing.

However, as this book emphasizes, reality is always more persuasive than theory.

On February 19, 2017, Jim opened an email from one "Trixie Boots" that read, in part: "I have been suffering from Lyme disease for about a decade and have tried many things for cure and symptomatic relief. I would like to discuss with you my current treatment that I am utilizing and get your opinion."

After trying many different therapies under different physicians with different theoretical orientations, and after hospitalizations and numerous visits to the ER, she was now microdosing and finding it beneficial. Jim asked her if she would write a description of her experience with the disease, including what had been tried and how microdosing had been helpful. The eight-page single-spaced document that she responded with presented a frightening odyssey. She had been treated by:

- physicians with no understanding of Lyme whatsoever
- many other specialists

- intensive bouts of medications, including multiple rounds of high-dose antibiotics and steroids (both of which are inherently dangerous)
- physicians who specialized in the treatment of Lyme

Although she had experienced transitory improvements in mental and physical symptoms, she had never approached what she called "normal." Before Lyme disease, she had been a high-functioning skilled athlete who'd completed her college education with high marks.

Here's an excerpt from her report:

> "I began microdosing after the last antibiotic run and began to feel 'normal.' I began to feel what I had used to feel as a normal person. Fatigue was absent, headaches disappeared, pain significantly lessened, circulation improved, and numbing in my hands and feet lessened. Something was happening on a neurological level that was somehow bringing all of these things into a state of harmony. Even though I have decreased blood flow in my frontal lobe which causes confusion, loss of memory, irritation, and focus issues, I seemed to experience a normal type of sensation cognitively. My heart which aches on a daily basis was not as painful day by day. Almost like it was not only relieving the symptoms but also having a lasting effect on the nervous system."

Her report concluded with a summary, "Microdosing: What does it do for me as a sufferer from Lyme and autoimmune issues?"

- "I no longer feel like a 500 lb. person is sitting on my body and restricting me from even moving a limb.
- Headaches which were daily and pounding and pressure in effect have completely dissipated.
- The pain that resonates through my joints, nerves, and muscles seems to relax upon dosing.

- Irritation and anxiety seem to disappear with dosing, however, when I take days off, it strikes back. But now I can recognize this behavior and try to defer it.
- Fatigue is nonexistent on this treatment. I think anyone with chronic fatigue should try this."

Over the years, Trixie continued to microdose and improve. She was able to hold down a job, and then an even better job. She had been married for six months when she had her initial ER visit, but the marriage didn't survive. She is now in a long-term relationship. She regularly communicates what she has learned to others who have persistent post-treatment Lyme, i.e., those whose course of antibiotics was either too late or ineffective.

The first published medical journal case of Lyme being treated with microdosing is similar to Trixie's story. In "The Effectiveness of Microdosed Psilocybin in the Treatment of Neuropsychiatric Lyme Disease: A Case Study,"[35] Daniel Kinderlehrer describes a forty-six-year-old man who "experienced the acute onset of fever, rigors, drenching sweats and myalgias." He tested positively for Lyme and was treated with doxycycline over the next ten months in combination with other antibiotics, stopping only when he felt "no apparent benefit." Over the next two decades he had "partial remissions and relapses. . . . The relapses lasted approximately 2 years."

At seventy years old, "he began microdosing psilocybin (desiccated whole mushrooms) 100 milligrams orally three times a week, increasing the dose to 125 milligrams after two weeks. Within two days, there was a noticeable improvement in mood. Within two weeks he was feeling completely well again. He has continued the regimen and two years later his depression and anxiety [as well as physical symptoms[36]] continue to be in remission."

A third case from a submitted report: a woman who had suffered from Lyme for five years, to the extent that she was intermittently totally debilitated, reported that microdosing psilocybin had been fundamental to her full recovery. We are in correspondence to get more details.

In addition, Baba Masha's book includes one case of Lyme, Report No. 730 (page 203): "I ate it [the *Amanita muscaria*] with pleasure as I clearly got better, and I felt all the symptoms receded. . . . By December I felt completely healthy. The tests showed that my blood was absolutely clean. Doctors could not understand what happened, but my blood was baby clean."[37]

For those suffering from long-lasting Lyme disease with multiple symptoms and ineffective treatment options, microdosing seems like a sensible and realistic option. We hope that cases like these encourage medical professionals to look more deeply into microdosing's possibilities. (Trixie's full report can be made available to serious medical professionals.)

Multiple Sclerosis (MS): A Case Study

Multiple sclerosis is a condition in which the immune system eats away at the protective covering of nerves, disrupting communication between the brain and the body. Symptoms may include vision loss, pain, fatigue, impaired coordination, and more.

Although MS is not fatal, there is no cure. The many treatments that are available either slow down the progression or diminish the severity of symptoms.

Usually diagnosed between the ages of twenty and fifty, it is most common in white people of Northern European descent, but occurs in most ethnic groups. It is three times more common among women. It is neither contagious nor inherited. Individuals with MS may suffer relapses (swift rise in symptoms) as in the case of the woman described below. Recovery from a relapse only returns someone back to their prior level of disability.

Case Study (edited for brevity and clarity)

"Dear Jim,

I have just watched your webinar. I have started typing to you a few times over the years to share my microdosing experience to contribute to your citizen science information. Finally, I'm writing.

I'll keep it short.

I was diagnosed with multiple sclerosis when I was 22 and at University. I have always, since I was a kid, suffered from terrible headaches and migraines. I am now 50 and am still walking about but with a cane for short distances or a walker for longer distances or more difficult terrain. I had a pretty bad relapse at the end of 2019 and had a course of heavy-duty steroids to dampen down the inflammation.

I decided to start microdosing LSD to see if I could calm my nervous system.

It's been nothing short of incredible:

I don't get headaches anymore.

I used to be plagued by cluster headaches and migraines.

I don't even get a hint of a headache anymore.

Incredible!

I didn't start microdosing thinking it would cure the MS. I was hoping it would settle my anxious baseline state and maybe help with fewer relapses. It has been so wonderful in doing both of those things.

The microdosing helps me to feel like everything isn't so hard, even though I wasn't even aware that things did feel hard (I hope that makes sense). I feel more connected to people and more at peace, possibly more content. Calmer. I have more really good days, as you would say. I do think I am probably anxious and get wound up easily and worry and fret. The microdosing settles all of that.

I'm hoping now that I can remain relapse free and start healing my damaged myelin [the insulating layer, or sheath, that forms around nerves].

All the best to you, Tom"

Jim heard back from her seven months later:

"Dear Jim,

I thought I'd write to you again after our correspondence last year. Two things you said resonated with me.

The first is the role microdosing has in neuroplasticity, growing new neural pathways. I think this has happened with me. I feel, after 3 years or so of following your protocol, not quite like a new person but certainly changed. Like there is an old me and a new me. I feel like my whole system, physical and psychological, is more in balance and in unity. It's a little easier to recognize when I'm feeling disordered and out of balance and then to bring myself back to normal. I'm possibly a bit more psychologically resilient.

The second point you made was eventually not needing to microdose. I'm not sure if I'm quite there yet, but over the past 6 months I haven't felt the need to keep up the dosage or frequency I used initially. I have reduced both and still feel well.

In the 7 months since our last correspondence, I remain free of any new MS symptoms and relapse free. My iPhone also informs me that I am walking more steps per day than I was this time last year!

My goal is to see some healing and improvement in my walking.

I also remain migraine and headache free!

I never thought I'd ever be able to say that.

All the very best to you.

Best wishes, Tom"

While this is our only report on this condition to date, it has already piqued the attention of researchers.

Palliative Care

My grandfather receives palliative care. He's an old hippie and asked me to get him some shrooms. Will they do him any good?

In some cases, he may feel better and be able to appreciate those who are with him. Individual dosing—tailored for each person—is important.

Palliative care is a "patient-centered model [that] prioritizes relief of suffering and tailors care to increase the quality of life for terminally ill patients."[38] It is not intended to extend a person's life but to maximize their comfort and capacity to benefit from the care of others.

Until very recently, there was no reported research on microdosing individuals with terminal illness. The first study is now underway in Canada. Here are three excerpts from the approved study description:

- "Interest in psychedelic medications has been rekindled by . . . two recent . . . trials [that] demonstrated rapid, clinically meaningful, and long-lasting reductions in depressed mood and/or anxiety symptoms and improvements in quality of life and death acceptance."
- "There is also evidence suggesting that psilocybin microdosing—taking sub-hallucinogenic doses continuously over longer time periods, rather than a one-time hallucinogenic dose—can improve mood and anxiety."
- "The goal of this trial is to demonstrate feasibility and preliminary measures of efficacy."[39]

The initial results (not yet published) are that, for some patients, microdoses given intermittently over a period of weeks substantially improved the quality of their lives. The newly developed protocol's dosage is to start low—with no effects reported—then raise the dose weekly until effects are experienced. The schedule for each week is:

- dose for two days
- take one day off
- dose for two days
- take two days off

When the study is over, those patients who reported sustained benefits will be given psilocybin to use at home or in medical facilities as long as they wish. As palliative care is such an important broad-based concern, any success here is likely to be followed up with additional efforts, studies, and citizen science reports.

A second study is also in the works. An approved double-blind study in New Zealand "is looking at the clinical possibilities of LSD with talk therapy for advanced cancer patients. . . . The microdosing trial is about treating the psychological problems people experience with late-term cancer, rather than the cancer itself."[40]

Pornography Addiction

I watch porn more than three hours a day. When I try to stop I feel miserable; when I watch, I feel trapped and ashamed. Can microdosing help here?

Addiction to pornography is a serious and growing problem.

Porn is a massive, highly profitable industry that shows no signs of diminishing (with AI-generated porn a whole new category). A review of the scientific and popular literature shows the most common concerns include reduced sexual activity among couples, a major increase in erectile dysfunction, and lowered sexual desire.

While there is a wide range of treatment options for porn, none seem especially effective. Treatments include: psychotherapy, behavioral therapy, couples therapy, sexual addiction therapy, support groups, twelve-step meetings, inpatient or outpatient treatment, and medications for co-occurring mental health and substance disorders (Miller, 2024).

The following single case suggests that microdosing might be considered as an alternative form of help:

> "I normally wouldn't share this, but I believe it's important and may possibly help others. I'm a 63-year-old male with high blood pressure and suffered a mild stroke a year and a half ago. I decided to microdose to see if it would help restore my cognitive abilities.
>
> While it did not seem to improve my memory or schedule management, the one thing I've noticed is that there's almost complete relief from a decades-long addiction to pornography. Over 30 years. At my worst point of several times a day, I could literally feel my brain calling for the chemical fix induced by the visual stimulation. I hated myself for my lack of self-control and my lack of integrity toward my loved ones, especially my wife.
>
> Since microdosing mushrooms at .20 grams every three days for the past three weeks, **the desire to use porn has completely vanished**. I think about it as a past event in my life. I did view it once on purpose to see what would happen and honestly, it just felt 'stupid and pointless.'
>
> Microdosing has released me from a life of shame and bondage; I had zero expectations that this was a possibility."

As with the often unexpected benefits that others have experienced in reducing their overconsumption of food, alcohol, or cannabis, microdosing may bring about a return to a healthier equilibrium in a way that is applicable to a wider variety of addictions, including ones like porn.

Post-Traumatic Stress Disorder (PTSD)

MDMA and PTSD are getting a lot of attention in the press, but can microdosing help people recover from PTSD as well?

Even without a clear understanding of the "why" or the "how," and even though it is little researched, we now know microdosing can help people recover.

PTSD, or post-traumatic stress disorder, is a mental health condition that develops after someone experiences a single traumatic event (or a series of them) in childhood or later. A wide range of traumatic experiences can cause PTSD.

Conventional therapy and current psychiatric medications are often unsuccessful in sufficiently alleviating symptoms for someone to feel normal. While the trauma(s) may have occurred even decades in the past, they are often easily "triggered"—that is, vividly and viscerally re-experienced in the present moment. This condition is extremely difficult to treat because almost any intervention, including psychotherapy, brings up such strong emotional reactions that it can be difficult for individuals to stay fully present and remain rational enough to work through the causes of what happened, and learn how to cope with their feelings.

For nearly ten years, we have recommended that individuals suffering from PTSD look to the growing body of successful MDMA interventions embedded in professional therapeutic protocols. Several years ago, the United States FDA "fast-tracked" MDMA-assisted therapy as a potentially innovative and successful PTSD treatment (only to have the first Lycos/MAPS application rejected in August 2024). As for microdosing, the general feeling had always been that it was simply not strong enough to be effective.

In June 2023, Jim's presentation notes for the huge MAPS (Multi-disciplinary Association for Psychedelic Studies[41]) Psychedelic Science conference in Denver repeated the above consensus notion: for something as difficult as PTSD, microdosing just wouldn't cut it.

However, literally the night before the presentation, a communication arrived from Richard Knowles, PhD, president of the Delos Psyche Research Group,[42] containing new information. The Delos group had put out a survey asking individuals who had treated their PTSD with microdosing if there had been any benefits. To our surprise—and contrary to our preconceptions—a number of individuals said microdosing had, indeed, substantially benefited them. One individual who responded to the survey wrote the following:

> "Prior to microdosing, my body would experience tonic immobility, which is relative to a seizure, followed by a tonic response: literally being frozen in the physical and mental realm of a trauma. Once microdosing, my body would stay relaxed, as my brain would recall intrusive thoughts, otherwise known as 'flashbacks.' I have safely mourned and processed 23 years of sexual, physical, emotional and verbal abuse from my primary caregivers, otherwise known as my 'parents.' I have not experienced tonic immobility after completing microdosing."

Another wrote:

> "Microdosing helps me feel more connected to my emotions and the world around me. This feeling of connection allows me to process and work through trauma and emotions in a healthy, therapeutic way that I haven't been able to achieve in the past."

A third added:

"Psilocybin has been the only thing I have come across to completely eliminate my intrusive thoughts. Without having to dose to the point of hallucinating, this substance has the most therapeutic effects with the least amount of adverse effects. I now take sertraline which does help, but it also comes with adverse effects. If I could be prescribed psilocybin, it would be the choice therapeutic drug overall for me."

The communications to the Delos Group also included a list of therapeutic benefits:

- Intrusive thoughts lessened
- Less hypervigilance
- Easier to relax
- Fewer physical symptoms of anxiety
- Less dissociation as well as a greater ability to stay in the present moment
- Lessened social anxiety related to trauma
- Many have quit their conventional antidepressant medication
- Reduced desire for substance use

Given microdosing's inherently high reward/risk ratio (that is, microdosing is extremely safe, far less costly, and does not need professional staff), it seems reasonable to suggest that individuals without access to MDMA-assisted therapy might benefit from microdosing.

We don't yet know to what degree it is helpful, or if there are any particular timing or dosing protocols that are especially valuable in the case of PTSD. If you have had any experience, successful or otherwise, using microdosing for PTSD, please complete the Delos Group's survey at delospsyche.org/survey.

Premenstrual Dysphoric Disorder (PMDD)

I've had PMDD for a few years, and my specialists haven't suggested anything that works. Has anyone tried microdosing? I'm desperate.

As this condition is generally not well understood, we'll take a more in-depth look. PMDD affects between 1 and 8 percent of women and is often treatment resistant. However, PMDD *is not a disease.* "PMDD appears to be a negative response to the normal fluctuations in female reproductive hormone levels . . . for most [women] hormone imbalance is not the cause of PMDD symptoms."[43] It is considered an extreme extension of PMS. Symptoms, which usually begin a week or more before menstruation and last for about two weeks out of every month, may include:

- **Emotional Symptoms:** Mood swings, tearfulness, increased sensitivity to rejection, irritability and anger, feelings of hopelessness and worthlessness, and self-deprecating thoughts.
- **Mental Challenges:** Loss of pleasure in previously pleasurable activities, feeling out of control, conflicts within otherwise good relationships, panic attacks, and most troubling, suicidal thoughts and plans.
- **Physical Changes:** Fatigue, inability to sleep or sleeping excessively, breast tenderness, joint or muscle pain, bloating or weight gain.[44]

One expert, Ally McHugh, described PMDD this way: "It impacts relationships, careers and can destroy a person's sense of identity and self-esteem. They spend half the month feeling disconnected, angry and lost, then often spend the other half feeling guilt and regret, having to put the pieces of their lives back together, then experiencing anxiety about the next cycle that will come around all too quickly."[45]

Given the remarkable span of PMDD symptoms, with people exhibiting symptoms of more than one condition, misdiagnosis often occurs.[46] There are several more or less successful treatments, many of which diminish in efficacy over time. These range from self-help (diet, exercise, psychotherapy) to taking SSRIs, neurosteroids, and bioidentical hormones.[47]

These next three reports are from women who had tried a number of other treatments prior to microdosing. (The first was in a public forum, the next two from personal correspondence with Jim.) We will hear from "Jess," who was just starting to microdose; "Naomi," who changed her dose and protocol as she entered menopause; and "Lucinda," who microdosed successfully over some years, followed by a few brief reports from other women.

After her first two microdoses, Jess wrote:

> "I am not even kidding you, those first two days, I said to my partner—I feel like I have like a serious brain injury and whatever I just consumed fit into a hole in my brain and made it function again. It was wild and I didn't expect it to be instantaneous at all. . . . I think it's letting me feel things that I would never let myself feel, so that's been really big. And honestly I want to feel those things and I want to unpack whatever it is that's keeping me stagnant and depressed."

Jess, three months later:

> "Overall, there's been a larger trend since I've been doing this over the last 3 months—my symptoms during the luteal phase have gone from two weeks to one week. I talked to my partner about it and asked—'Am I imagining this?!'"[48]

Naomi is a professional health worker in Scandinavia. In 2019 she wrote:

"My doctor suspected PMDD and got me started on an SSRI (citalopram) the last week before my menstruations about 2.5 years ago (my hormonal levels are still normal). . . . The PMDD improved a little until this spring/summer when the brain fog, depressive feeling and fatigue got really bad. It really made my life suck, and my working capacity was really low. Since I'm self-employed, this was serious!

In my desperation I took my first dose of a microdose (LSD) on August 1st (still on the SSRI). What a game changer! I have not felt better in years. . . .

My quality of life has changed completely!!!

My happy mood is back, my energy level is back (the brain fog, fatigue and irritability have vanished), my working capacity is normalized, I'm less introverted, more positive and outgoing. I can also see it in my income!"

In 2021 she reported:

"It goes very well. I have now been microdosing nonstop for 1.5 years (since August 2019). I have really come to appreciate the use and effect of microdosing. I just turned 50, and menopause has hit me hard with hot flashes and bad sleep.

Just before Christmas, I stopped using SSRIs completely. I had been alternating microdoses and SSRIs every other 5th day (2.5 days between each dose) . . . and I didn't get any abstinence symptoms. I noticed that I still needed my microdose . . . AND . . . I couldn't use it every fifth day, because the fatigue, irritability, mood swings and bad brain fog were reappearing. Instead, I shortened the intervals and now take my microdose every 3rd or 4th day (which equals 2 times a week; Wednesday and Saturday or Sunday).

Actually, I feel the effect of the microdose is even better, clearer and cleaner—without the SSRI. My mood, spirit, energy and cognition are supergood—even though some low days come around every now and then, but these I can live with! . . .

I'll guess I use 1/20th of a full dose now. With 1/20th, I feel the effect as a lifted mood, good spirit and an inner flow of positive energy. For how long I will continue with microdosing, I don't know. But I will not quit in the foreseeable future."

In 2023 she added:

"So . . . I continued with my microdose regimen (every 3–4 days) up until 2023. I'm now way into menopause and respond very well to hormone replacement therapy for typical problems such as hot flashes, dry mucous membranes and bad sleep. . . .

I have much energy and good working capacity, my menopause is stable/ongoing, and the need for microdosing is not that pronounced. I do it in periods where I feel I need a little extra energy kick or when I just need to be lifted to normal energy levels and wellbeing. . . . When I'm not tired or exhausted from work, but feeling normal, a microdose on such a day can really boost my energy level and mood. My previous, almost chronic, fatigue and brain fog are more or less gone."[49]

Lucinda is the executive assistant to the president of a large multinational nonprofit. In 2020 she wrote:

"In 2017, I was diagnosed with PMDD and in September I was prescribed an SSRI to be taken during the luteal phase. It made me emotionally numb, which was a nice change, but after a couple of months, I was back in the depths of darkness. Shortly after, I started the microdosing. That was in December of 2017. I have only been microdosing during my luteal phase. I dose before bed on day one of ovulation, then take two days off, dose on the third day before bed, then take three days off. I repeat this until the first day of my menstruation, at which point I stop until ovulation occurs again. I have been dosing during my luteal phase like this ever since. It has changed my life in the most profound way; I am the most mentally, emotionally, and financially stable I have ever been."

In 2023 she added:

"I'm still microdosing for PMDD. Next month, it will be 6 years! (I have tracked my moods/symptoms with a PMDD tracking app since I started microdosing, and use a period tracking app to determine ovulation.)"[50]

Finally, here are a few brief reports from the Reddit "psychedelic women" thread:[51]

- "Microdosing during PMS week eliminates my suicidal ideation and wanting to leave my family. I 100% recommend it. Am finally off birth control and antidepressants after 15 years."
- "I started MDing about 5 months ago. It's helped tremendously. I still experience those feelings, but I don't identify with them . . . I observe and release them. I'm also able to experience glimpses of actual joy."
- "For me, microdosing just makes me feel normal."

Conclusion: Each case reviewed here addresses a different constellation of symptoms, with microdosing leading to differing levels of relief. For some, microdosing has been a genuine magic bullet. For others, it has been very helpful, even when not providing full remission.

Resource: DysphoricProject.org. This site is specifically for women with PMDD and embraces helping them with microdosing. **A number of reports in this section came from this site.** As one woman on the site said in a long interview about her improvements:

"Just do it. Rather than wasting the time, do it over not doing it. If there are changes or adjustments that need to be made, they can be made later. There's so little risk with a microdose and there's so much benefit that can come from it—we're really doing a disservice to ourselves [by continuing to just live with PMDD]."

Premenstrual Syndrome (PMS)

I heard Doctor Fadiman give a talk at Breaking Convention where he told a story about PMS and microdosing. I don't recall if the upshot was "yes," "no," or "take your chances."

The definition of PMS is simple enough: "Many women feel physical or mood changes during the days before menstruation. When these symptoms happen month after month, and they affect a woman's normal life, they are known as premenstrual syndrome (PMS)."[52]

Jim wrote back to the questioner as follows:

Your memory almost got it right. I did give a talk at the Breaking Convention conference about microdosing, but said nothing about PMS. However, I did ask the people there to write me about their own experiences. A couple of months later, I got the following email from a woman who introduced herself as an art historian:

"I know I owe you a letter about my microdosing, and I thought this would interest you: my periods have always been painful, but when I was microdosing as you suggested, I had my first normal one. Just thought you'd like to know."

Jim asked her some basic questions: What was her dose? What substance? Which protocol, if any? And when during each month was she microdosing? She replied that she had only microdosed for that one month, and not again. Jim remembers her last sentence very clearly:

"My periods are now normal. You have changed my life. Thank you."

When Jim shared this story with Sophia Korb, she said their reports included three or four women who found their PMS symptoms pretty much went away while microdosing. None of them said they used it for only one month. Sophia then went and talked to a PMS researcher. All she was told was that there were a lot of reasons why people might have started having normal periods, and that she had no idea why microdoses would help.

What we can say, and what fits in with what else we know, is that to the extent PMS is a dysregulation of the changing hormone levels women go through during their period, microdosing can help by moving a woman's system toward normal.

Schizophrenia

Are microdoses off-limits for anyone who is or has been schizophrenic? Could it be helpful?

Background: Schizophrenia is a disorder that affects a person's ability to think, feel, and behave clearly. It is characterized by thoughts or experiences that seem out of touch with reality, often including delusions and hallucinations. High doses of any psychedelic are contraindicated, especially outside a safe therapeutic environment. For a condition often described as being "in a different reality," the reality-altering effects of high doses are unlikely to be helpful.

Before the importance of set and setting was understood, high doses of psychedelics, given in sterile clinical settings, led to what appeared to be classic psychotic or schizophrenic episodes. For a while, doses were even given to medical personnel so they could have a better understanding of the hellish inner world of their patients. One of the suggested names for psychedelics at that time was "psychotomimetic"— mimicking psychosis.

Later, the first research stressing a safe and comfortable set and setting—treating chronic treatment-resistant alcoholics in Canada— showed highly positive effects. A different researcher, saying he was attempting to replicate the experiment, gave similar alcoholics similar doses, but left them alone and literally shackled to hospital beds in an empty room for the duration of the treatment. He reported this was not successful, establishing—perhaps unintentionally—that "psychedelic-assisted therapy" was beneficial, while "psychotomimetic treatment" was not.

Current psychiatric information states that treatment can help, but schizophrenia can't be cured. Online resources suggest that 25 percent of individuals recover on their own and that medication is helpful for many others. It is a condition that is not well understood, in part because of the enormous variation of symptoms.

We were not planning to include any discussion of schizophrenia, but our mind was changed by a report and subsequent publication by Mark Haden, the prior director of MAPS Canada. In the initial 2019 report, Haden wrote:

> I ran into an individual, who has schizophrenia and . . . over a
> multi-decade process, he figured out that high dosages of any-
> thing like cannabis or psychedelics are really horrible for him.
> They destabilize him and his life goes completely off the rails.
> But what he discovered is a very, very small dose of either
> LSD or mushrooms seems to change the voices . . . he has in
> his head that are normally negative, judgmental, destructive,

nasty voices that are very condemning of him. When he takes
a psychedelic *micro-dose, a tiny, tiny [amount]*, the voices are
still there, but they change and they become very loving and
positive to him.[53]

After learning that a low dose was used successfully when high doses
had been damaging, Haden had earlier noted that "It seems to be *there is
a threshold in which it turns from positive to negative.*" (Haden interview;
emphasis in original.)

Haden's 2023 article explored this history as well as revised contemporary reports and studies. The central finding of Haden and his
co-authors was that "while psychedelics are not a panacea, there are
circumstances where they have been shown to be helpful for individuals with schizophrenia."[54] This conclusion was specific: "The authors
of this paper tentatively observe that a low dose or a microdose of a
psychedelic may be a possible treatment for the negative symptoms of
schizophrenia."

As of now, there are no known understood causes of schizophrenia, only possible genetic, environmental, and traumatic ones. In other
words, we don't know much, and it will probably ultimately be seen as
a collection of symptoms, including the puzzling ones described here.
As is true of other disorders described in this book, it is likely that low
doses are relatively safe and may lead to lessened symptoms.

Sleep

Can microdosing help improve my sleep?

If microdosing generally acts as a stimulant, how can it possibly
improve sleep? We consistently read that microdosing boosts alert-
ness, enables longer creative work sessions, improves strength and
running speed, and activates and enhances other abilities as well.

That's why the rule of thumb* is to take a microdose before ten or eleven in the morning so that it won't keep you up past a healthy (for you) bedtime.

Therefore, it seemingly made no sense when a trustworthy organization like the Microdosing Institute of the Netherlands recommended taking microdoses at night for sleep disorders.

Perhaps *microdoses weren't actually a stimulant.* Admittedly, microdosing often does do much of what a stimulant does. And, indeed, some people take microdoses instead of Adderall or other amphetamine products, reporting they get similar effects but without the inevitable crash.

Suppose, instead, we think of microdosing as a *general system enhancer.* While awake, it improves waking physiology and behaviors. At night, it improves sleep physiology and behaviors. It also makes sense of why we have so many reports not only of longer and deeper sleep and people feeling more rested but of "nicer dreams" that are less disturbed, anxious, or sad.

For example, one spontaneous report came from a healthy sixty-one-year-old man whose home was rented by Big Think for an interview with Jim. The man wore an Oura ring that precisely tracks how long he sleeps and the quality of that sleep. The man initially told Jim that he was interested in psychedelics, and while he hadn't yet taken any, he was intending to. A bit later, he offered that he actually *had* microdosed for the first time the night before. Then he said, "What I saw when I looked at my sleep record today is that I'd slept almost *double* the number of minutes in deep sleep that's usual for me."

As for "hard data," a randomized placebo-controlled 2023 study used sleep monitors to measure exactly how much participants actually

---

*One exception to this rule of thumb may be *Amanita muscaria,* which has an increasing reputation for use either earlier in the day or as a sleep enhancer about half an hour before bed. A general "nightcap" protocol, applicable to all types of microdosing substances, is described in chapter 2.

slept during each night of the few weeks of the study. It followed the Fadiman protocol—after microdosing on day one, participants did not microdose on days two or three. According to the study's abstract:

> 80 healthy adult male volunteers received a 6-week course of either LSD (10 µg) or placebo with doses self-administered every third day. . . . Data from 3231 nights of sleep showed that *on the night after microdosing, participants in the LSD group slept an extra 24.3 minutes per night . . .* compared to placebo—with no reductions of sleep observed on the dosing day itself. There were no changes in the proportion of time spent in various sleep stages or in participant physical activity.[55] (Emphasis added.)

This unexpected finding—that participants slept almost twenty-five minutes longer on the second night after microdosing—led to the study being widely reported in the press.

We know from many individual reports that people often report improved sleep, and sometimes primarily microdose for sleep and are satisfied with the results. It seems safe to say that microdosing, properly undertaken, makes healthier sleep more likely, including more sleep in general and likely more deep sleep.

Stroke

Seven years ago my husband had a major stroke. He suffers from many limitations. Could microdosing make a difference?

Strokes are the leading cause of serious long-term disability and the fifth leading cause of death in adults in the US. Strokes occur when blood flow to the brain is blocked; within minutes, brain cells begin to die. Medical intervention can stop the damage and rehabilitation can help restore lost functioning.

With some conditions, like headaches and depression, we know a lot. With others, like stroke, we are just at the beginning.

Here are a few reports from Reddit:

- "I started microdosing a few years after my stroke and it has helped immensely. I combine either with lion's mane and niacin (Stamets stack) or an anti-stress combo with theanine and ashwagandha. It has helped my energy and mood."[56]
- "[A] close friend of mine suffered brain damage from a stroke. Drawn from his experience . . . psilocybin, even when only microdosed, helped him A LOT to recover."[57]
- "I notice improvements across the board with .15–.2g of daily psilocybin. I also see benefit with my hypertension—a 3-day MD run is worth 10 points lower BP, all diet-related issues being equal. I'm personally convinced my stroke recovery has been significantly aided by the improved mood, verbal ability, and perhaps neural plasticity improvements of MD'ing."[58]

The following report is by a son about his father's stroke. He found that psilocybin microdosing had produced "mostly positive or neutral results." After giving his dad 0.5 grams of psilocybin and going to a movie, he wrote:

"Excellent results! My dad was focused on the movie, and was emotional and laughing at appropriate scenes. . . . He even said that he felt 'pretty good' after the movie, which he hadn't said in years."[59]

While his father found some benefit in psilocybin microdosing, his son also found that "ultimately, my dad's post-stroke psychological issues, such as anger, depression, agitation, and obsessive compulsion were *better soothed by marijuana.*"[60] (Emphasis in original.)

We conclude with a case report from a woman whose husband had been a professional musician, an outgoing social man who traveled and played for many years. After his stroke at age seventy he was unable to play, initially unable to walk, and had speech and other difficulties. Between conventional rehabilitation and alternative medical support, he regained most of his speech, walked slowly with a cane, and could get upstairs . . . but with difficulty. Over the next six years he made additional improvements, but was still far from recovered. Jim tells the story from there:

> I met with his wife, who gave me the above information and asked if microdosing might help. At that time, there was very little information about microdosing for physical health problems, but it often seemed to reduce pain and improve mood. She decided to go ahead, and her husband agreed.
>
> After several weeks, she reported that he was more social, sleeping better, in better spirits, and seemed to be walking better. Her friends and his physician noticed the improvements. He was also drinking less, which had been a major concern. Over the next month, he continued to improve, including climbing stairs more easily.
>
> To her surprise, he said he wanted to visit friends who lived in Mexico. He had not traveled for years. She said she would be very happy to travel with him, but it would take several weeks to reschedule her clients. He said he wanted to go sooner, and he would go on his own.
>
> After considerable hesitation, and only after his doctor's agreement, she agreed. While the actual travel was not easy, he did it on his own. He was met at the airport and taken care of by his friends.
>
> After a few days, he phoned her. "I'm doing well, and I'm taking a daily short walk with our friends."
>
> He called again several days later. "I'm no longer using my cane."

Substantial recovery from a debilitating condition—seven years later—is worth noting.

Baba Masha reports on seventeen people with strokes who microdosed *Amanita muscaria*. Six experienced positive results, two had negative results, and nine had no results. One of the positive reports reads in part: "My friend treated her mother (eighty-six years) with AM microdosing after a stroke. She eventually recovered very quickly, now she walks and speaks well" (Masha, p. 224).

Baba Masha writes: "The effects of . . . microdosing on stroke . . . require a closer, more detailed consideration of the effects and severity of the condition. In the framework of the project as a preliminary study, the results are enough to warrant such further investigation."[61] We agree. Along these lines, Algernon Pharmaceuticals began Phase I safety trials in 2023. It "eventually hopes to use small, non-hallucinogenic doses of DMT—DMT microdoses in other words—to treat stroke patients."[62]

Some stroke patients have had remarkable improvements from microdosing. At the very least, based on the individual particulars and severity of a stroke victim's situation, it may be worth considering microdosing as an optional addition to other modes of recovery.

Stuttering

I stutter. Paul Stamets cured his with a lot of mushrooms. That's too scary for me. Can I start with a microdose?

According to the US National Institutes of Health, "Stuttering is a speech disorder characterized by repetition of sounds, syllables, or words; prolongation of sounds; and interruptions in speech known as blocks. An individual who stutters exactly knows what he or she would like to say but has trouble producing a normal flow of speech."

- Boys are 2 to 3 times as likely to stutter as girls and as they get older this gender difference increases. . . .

- The precise mechanisms that cause stuttering are not understood. . . .
- Although there is currently no cure for stuttering, there are a variety of treatments.[63]

As for Paul Stamets, the remarkable story he tells includes an unusual setting and a strongly focused intention. As a teenager, he stuttered severely. At one point in his life he obtained a small bag of mushrooms. After eating them—his first psychedelic experience—he climbed a tree. Soon after that came a furious rainstorm, windstorm, and—most frightening to Paul—lightning storm. As he hung on to the tree for hours, he kept repeating to himself the words "stop stuttering now." When he came down from the tree, he was able to speak without a stutter.[64]

The next day, a girl he liked passed by. His old self would never have spoken to her because he would have stuttered and felt ashamed. The post-psychedelic Paul said hello. She responded warmly. His life was never the same, with his speech showing no sign of his previous stuttering.*

We have three reports in our files.

1. A young man, in Paul Stamets fashion, decided that he would stop stuttering. During a solo LSD session (not his first), he spent several hours sitting on the end of a diving board strongly telling himself that his stuttering would stop. No storm. No lightning. However, over the next few weeks, his stuttering diminished to very close to normal speech.

2. A male college student was intensely aware that he felt that his stuttering made any kind of normal social life—especially dating—almost impossible. He began microdosing and almost immediately was able to speak normally for several hours and even went to parties successfully. He became so fascinated

---

*Individuals who have worked intensely for years to gain control over their stuttering often retain a particular speech pattern that speech therapists easily recognize. For example, when President Biden sometimes stumbled over a word, although his opponents suggested it was his age, it was actually the residue of his stuttering.

with this shift in speech, although it did not seem to last, that he changed his major and graduated in speech therapy with an emphasis on stuttering. He continued to microdose on social occasions and also finds cannabis very helpful.

3. A man in his late thirties, who had tried various forms of speech training, was working intensely with a particular method that he was told needed to be constantly maintained to be useful. While he was microdosing correctly with a protocol, he found some, but not much, improvement. He felt it was likely that the speech method he practiced may have limited the value of the microdosing.

We know that stuttering is more likely to increase under stress, and there are particular situations, such as speaking on the phone or saying one's own name, that can be extremely difficult. Stutterers can often be perfectly fluid when speaking or singing along with others, or reciting or acting memorized speech.

While microdosing may be useful in reducing social anxiety and the tension around specific activities, at this time there is not enough evidence to recommend it specifically for alleviating stuttering. We'll let you know if more reports come in.

Traumatic Brain Injury (TBI)

I smashed into a rock downhill skiing. Serious brain injury. After two years of rehabilitation, they said that's all the healing that's going to happen, but I'm still pretty much disabled. I read about a hockey player who got better with mushrooms. Any truth to it?

Yes, it's true.

Traumatic brain injury (TBI) happens when a sudden external physical assault damages the brain. It is one of the most common causes of disability and death in adults. TBI is a broad term that describes a vast array of injuries that happen to the brain. The damage can be focal (confined to one area of the brain) or diffuse (happens in more than one area of the brain).[65]

Some mild brain injuries seem to disappear after a few months, but other more severe injuries can result in permanent disability, even after extensive rehabilitation. Symptoms can include cognitive deficits, motor deficits, perceptual or sensory deficits, communication and language deficits, inability to drive a car, social difficulties, regulatory disturbances, dizziness, loss of bladder and bowel control, personality changes, and cursing or inappropriate sexual behavior. It's a depressingly long list. (Perhaps this is why the National Football League has paid out more than $1.25 billion to more than 1,700 former pro football athletes for traumatic brain injuries.[66])

Before turning to a case study of a hockey player's recovery from TBI, let's take this opportunity to describe the uneven process that begins with a first report on microdosing helping a condition and over time develops into fuller understanding and more effective usage.

At the 2017 MAPS[67] conference in Oakland, after Jim and Sophia presented results from their first seven hundred microdosing reports, people there wanted to share their experiences. Among them was a young man who had been almost totally incapacitated after a skull fracture from a car accident. He said that two years of rehabilitation had been helpful, but he still suffered from painful headaches. Microdosing to become less depressed, he found it also stopped the headaches.

Later that same evening, a middle-aged man, formerly a jump rope athlete, spoke with Jim. He told him that after his TBI, he could no longer do the jumps he'd done before. However, in the last six months he'd been microdosing, and while he wasn't as skilled as he'd once been, he was able to do most of the difficult jumps again.

At that time, there was little understanding and no formal research about any aspect of microdosing. No one even considered the possibility of it helping physical conditions. What interest there was, was in its effects on mental states. There were no coaches, no groups, and the Microdosing Institute in Holland was barely a year old.

With so much going on—the helter-skelter conference of stimulus overload, interview requests, documentaries, presentations, and meeting with friends—Jim didn't recognize how extraordinary the two stories were . . . and almost forgot about them.

In 2021, Adam Bramlage, a microdosing coach with a number of professional athlete clients, introduced Jim to Daniel Carcillo, a former professional hockey player who was retired at age thirty because of brain concussions. At that point, with the current psychedelic revival in its first flowering and hundreds of companies pitching psychedelic-related drugs worldwide, microdosing was still barely being noticed.

After conventional rehabilitation had been unsuccessful, Daniel benefited enormously from high-dose psychedelic therapy followed by microdosing.

Before working with psychedelics, he had been planning suicide. But when Jim met him, he was running a startup, including setting up research projects with universities developing new therapeutic models, and displayed no symptoms of mental or physical disorganization or dysfunction. If using psychedelics to treat traumatic brain injury needed a poster child, Daniel was it.

From interviews with Daniel and from detailed descriptions of athletes working with Adam, there is every reason to support integrating microdosing into any traumatic brain injury treatment as soon as possible. While this may seem like a radical possibility, it seems that microdosing *actually supports healing of damaged areas of the brain.*

We have one last report, from another hockey player, also retired due to concussions. After having completed rehabilitation, he spent most of his time in a darkened bedroom because that's where his headaches were least likely to become too painful. After working with Adam, and using both microdosing and other functional mushrooms, not only could he leave his room but he resumed a normal enough life to get engaged and married. At some point in his healing, he realized he had no more need for microdosing.

Varicella-Zoster Virus (Shingles)

My doctor says it will pass, but right now, I can barely sleep because of the pain. And I hate and fear opiates. Will a microdose or even a higher dose be of any use?

Shingles is a viral infection caused by the varicella-zoster virus—the same virus that causes chickenpox. If you've had chickenpox, the virus remains in your body for the rest of your life. Years later, if the virus reactivates, it can cause shingles, usually appearing as a single stripe of blisters on one side of the torso. Shingles can appear anywhere, however, including inside your mouth or on your genitals. The pain can last weeks, even after all the blisters are gone. It is a nonfatal, but nasty, condition.

Shingles is more common in older adults and those with weakened immune systems. It's important to note that like chickenpox, it is contagious, but it can only be spread to people who have never had chickenpox and have not been vaccinated for it.[68]

Jim received an email from a man in Namibia* with a terrible case of shingles. After several weeks of increasing pain, he reported that no matter what position he slept in, the pressure on his skin was so painful it woke him up.

Friends he knew in the capital suggested he try a mushroom. He had no prior experience with any psychedelic. He wrote: "Within 45 minutes my pain was gone, really gone! That was two weeks ago. Now if I feel a tingling, like the pain coming back, I just take a little mushroom and it goes away."

A very excited Jim reached out to his collaborator, Sophia Korb. After reaching her upon her return from an international psychedelics conference in Prague, her response was: "What an amazing coincidence. Twice

---

*Namibia is the world's thirty-fourth largest country. Located in southern Africa, it is (after Mongolia) the second least densely populated country in the world (2.7 inhabitants per square kilometer, 7.0 per square mile).

at the conference, two women approached me, threw their arms around me, and wept, thanking us for our work. In both cases, microdosing had relieved their husbands' painful shingles."

However, Jim and Sophia misinterpreted the initial reports, believing that microdoses could *heal* shingles.

Over the next several years, when asked about unusual results, Jim would include the Namibia story, saying how remarkable it was that a microdose could affect the shingles virus. So, it seemed fortuitous when a friend arrived from overseas with shingles.

The friend had planned a several-week pleasure trip to the US but was instead too miserable with shingles to pursue anything. When she was awake, she was crumpled up with pain, and when she was asleep, her pain frequently woke her. A friend of Jim's had some psilocybin microdose capsules mixed with other mushrooms. Jim suggested she try them. Within a short time, to her amazement, she felt almost no pain and was able to sit and stand normally.

However, within about eight hours, the pain returned with full force. She took a second dose, with similar results. Eight hours later, awakened from sleep with pain, she took a third dose and slept through the night. On the second day, the pain-free period extended to nine hours between doses, and after several days, to twelve hours. Her pain continued to diminish over the next week, so she was able to visit friends and travel back to her home in South America carrying microdoses with her.

It was unlikely that the microdose interacted with the virus. But, perhaps by providing her body and immune system with general support, the microdose helped her successfully deal with the pain. It's unclear whether the diminishing pain over time was part of the natural cycle of shingles, or whether the support of microdoses enabled her immune system to continue to improve her capacity to cope with the symptoms.

We can suggest that *while microdosing is likely to reduce pain from shingles, the usual protocols may not be effective, and doses should be taken as soon as the pain reappears.*

One final surprise: after the second dose, she reported feeling better than she had in years. A woman in her midsixties, she had been beset by chronic multi-symptom conditions plus pain and scarring from an operation in her twenties. While she functioned well in the world, she acknowledged she was usually in some pain. No longer in pain from the shingles, she insisted that she was far more comfortable and flexible in her body than she had been for a very long time. She had been a dancer, but hadn't danced for at least the last 15 years. She then did a little happy dance, before standing on one foot, easily balancing—which had been impossible for her for years.

During the period while microdosing, she reported feeling feminine for the first time in years, wanting to dress and look prettier. She was indeed more animated, with more color in her face and eyes that were bright. She seemed much younger. After returning to South America, she wrote that these "feminine" changes seemed permanent. However, like the original African correspondent, from time to time she would feel the beginnings of shingles pain and needed to microdose.

The way she used microdosing for shingles *did not fit into any of the prescribed protocols and did not prevent shingles from continuing to be a problem.* While we emphasize the necessity for protocols with time off between doses, there are situations, like this one, that call for totally different dosing regimens. As for her increased vitality, it remains to be investigated but is consonant with many microdosers reporting less depression, more happiness, and healthier habits.

Note: The original question also asked about high doses. While it's highly likely that during a session pain would be reduced or not experienced, it's not a good idea to attempt a high dose when so physically debilitated. Also, since the pain is likely to return—as it does for microdosing—it's probably not worth the time or risk of a high-dose session.

[6]

Science and History

When the data and the anecdotes disagree,
the anecdotes are usually right.
And it doesn't mean you just slavishly go follow
the anecdotes then. It means you go examine
the data. It's usually not that the data is being
mis-collected, it's usually that you're not
measuring the right thing.
—Jeff Bezos[1]

Much more could be said about both the science and history of microdosing than this book can cover. Even as we are diligently working to wrap up this book, new scientific studies and real-world developments—ones that one day may very well be seen as historic—keep occurring.

Our goal in this chapter is therefore modest: to bring together and present enough of the science and history for you to more easily see the big picture for yourself, ask the right questions, and make the best choices for you and your loved ones.

Research Rising

Given all the excitement about microdosing, why isn't there more research?

Modern microdosing is less than fifteen years old, with psychedelics research overall "off the table" for a few decades before that. Even so, there are close to fifteen hundred microdosing studies listed in PubMed, the US National Institutes of Health's online publication database, with more added each year. In 2024 alone, there were close to two hundred new studies in the first quarter.

Why hasn't there been more definitive research by now? Professor David Nutt, a well-regarded British neuropsychopharmacologist, gives a compelling answer:

> Until the past couple of years, there were almost no formal studies (there are still very few). This isn't surprising. In countries and states where psychedelics are illegal—most of them—a single molecule is as illegal as a kilo, so there are the same barriers to research if you want to use only tiny amounts in a study as there are with larger-dose studies: namely, stigma and reputational risk, very high costs, and safety- and ethics-related administrative red tape.
>
> At Imperial College, we managed to get ethical permission and some funding from the Beckley Foundation for an LSD microdosing study. But we couldn't afford to do it. The legal requirements, and the safety rules imposed by the ethics committee, were the same as if we were using a full dose: locking drugs in the safe, giving the drug only in [the] hospital, keeping the participant in and under observation for a whole day. The difference is that for microdosing, you have to dose each subject multiple times, and as each would have required a hospital admission this made the study prohibitively expensive.[2]

Given these obstacles, Nutt continues, most academic microdosing studies have been survey-based, "with people using their own drugs in a naturalistic setting."[3]

More research is underway and will continue to increase as microdosing's popularity grows. Let's review the best-known and largest microdosing survey and what it showed.

Microdose.me Survey Results

What was shown by the big Microdose.me survey studies?

Beginning in 2020, more than eight thousand people contributed data to an online app-based study by Microdose.me. (As of this writing, you can still participate at Microdose.me.) Two articles have been published in *Scientific Reports—Nature*; the first, titled "Adults Who Microdose Psychedelics Report Health Related Motivations and Lower Levels of Anxiety and Depression Compared to Non-microdosers," was 2021's third-most downloaded paper from that journal.[4]

The Beckley Foundation, a longtime psychedelic research center, summarized the study:

> Participants were asked whether or not they were currently
> microdosing, and if they had any psychological, mental health
> or addiction concerns. Mental health was assessed using the
> DASS-21 scale, to obtain measures of depression, anxiety and
> stress levels. . . . When these scales were compared between
> microdosers and non-microdosers reporting mental health
> concerns, it was found that microdosers exhibited lower scores
> on all three, indicating that microdosing may be beneficial for
> treating certain mental health conditions.[5]

The Beckley report noted "another interesting observation . . . of lower alcohol and tobacco use among the microdosing group. This finding is consistent with previous studies having reported healthier lifestyles in psychedelic users."[6]*

---

*Throughout this book we make reference to how microdosing helps some people reduce or quit the use of cigarettes and tobacco products. Here is a typical report:

"October this year will mark three years [since microdosing] free of cigarettes for me. I've never once had a craving or had the feeling I might some day go back to being a smoker. Oftentimes when people quit smoking, the cravings never subside . . . it's quite the opposite for me."

One of its authors, Joseph Rootman, further explained:

Among individuals reporting mental health concerns, the microdosing group reported lower levels of depression, anxiety and stress than their non-microdosing peers. These findings align with the idea that many microdosers are engaging in the practice with the intent of managing mental health and is suggestive of the relative safety of microdosing among individuals with mental health concerns.[7]

Rootman also made an important methodological observation with broad long-term implications:

Researchers seeking to investigate the effects of these substances in the laboratory are presented with the challenge of replicating natural psychedelic settings. Considering these challenges, it is likely that the future of psychedelic research will be flexible and integrate a variety of methodological approaches. . . . Our successful recruitment and engagement of thousands of participants . . . illustrates the promise ahead for the field of psychedelic research more broadly. . . . Innovations in technology have substantially reduced barriers to engaging participants in research studies.[8]

The second article on the Microdose.me study concluded "greater observed improvements in mood and mental health at one month relative to non-microdosing controls. . . . Comparisons of microdosers to non-microdosers indicated greater improvements among microdosers . . . within *Depression, Anxiety,* and *Stress* . . . microdose-related reductions in depression were stronger among females than males . . . microdosers exhibited greater increases in positive mood . . . and larger decreases in negative mood over the study duration."[9]

Future psychedelic research (especially on microdosing) will continue to include observations by citizen scientists as a key component. That is where modern microdosing began, and given the growth in survey study technology as well as the general growth of interest in microdosing, we can expect that especially as new medical conditions and positive uses are discovered, they will originate from citizen scientists.

> All cases are unique,
> and very similar to others.
> —T. S. Eliot

Contemporary Observational Science

How does the science of microdosing, including relying on firsthand reports, sync up with the way science works?

What we now call "the scientific revolution" began more than 350 years ago with the founding of the Royal Society of London, with its founding motto *Nullius in verba,* which translates as "Nothing on authority." Historian Mike Jay describes it this way:

> It announced a new way of thinking that came to dominate the scientific revolution: Classical and scholastic authority could prove apocryphal. Only direct evidence, generated by experiment and first-person observation, revealed scientific truth.
>
> Evidence was everything, and leading scientists of the era . . . developed a system for classifying it. Qualities such as size, shape, or weight, which were directly measurable, were referred to as "primary" evidence. Texture, taste, or feelings that described human sensation and responses were

considered "secondary." While primary evidence was easier to collect and test, sensation and perception were considered legitimate fields of inquiry, and certain classes of data could only be demonstrated by self-experiment.[10]

We now say "objective "and "subjective" instead of "primary" and "secondary," but the basic distinctions remain. Observations of internal states and hard-to-measure physical changes taken together—especially when collated and considered by a "community of the qualified"*— can offer us unique insights into our own and others' experiences.

Many thousands of microdosing reports from around the world have allowed us to predict findings for a wide variety of physical and mental conditions, as well as ways of enhancing capabilities, capacities, and wellness. In contrast, modern scientific methodology—which relies on distilling observations into numerical data—did not and could not have replicated the large pool of observations presented throughout this book.

At a recent psychedelics conference in Exeter, England, a prominent researcher gave his conclusion about the most current set of microdose studies:

> The more and better controlled the research is, the lower the effects are, with the consequence that the most elaborate methodologically sound research gives the impression that there is no effect.[11]

This researcher recognized that the closer microdosing experiments approach experimental perfection (randomized, double-blind, placebo-

---

*Philosopher Ken Wilber defined "inter-subjective hermeneutical verification" as the process by which a panel of those selected from a "community of the qualified"—for example, a panel of Zen masters evaluating a beginner's progress—are able to engage and come to agreement to evaluate things that are completely subjective (secondary evidence), including most of what's important about microdosing.

controlled, etc.), the less they show anticipated microdosing effects (factoring out expectations).* This is also exactly what we have predicted. What a relief to see it admitted.

There could be *no more conclusive way of demonstrating that the wrong tool, methodology, or mode of analysis is often used to study microdosing.* As the psychologist Abraham Maslow said, "it is tempting, if the only tool you have is a hammer, to treat everything as if it were a nail."[12]

Looking at the cases reported throughout this book, selected from many others, we can say that *the closer one gets to personal observations from real-world situations, the more impressive the data becomes.*

Often referred to as "the gold standard" for research, the idealized experimental method (double-blind, placebo-controlled, etc.) may still be the best tool for comparing effects between closely related substances or interventions, like measuring the effectiveness of a new antidepressant against an older one. The reality is that this specific methodology is baked into the US Food and Drug Administration's regulations for seeking the right to sell drugs.[†] It has never been workable for psychedelic studies, as even for microdoses, the "blind" is almost always ineffective.[‡]

To understand why any of this matters, let's return to the history of science.

---

*Such a conclusion—that studies that meet ever-stricter experimental criteria increasingly show a lack of evidence—assumes that standard scientific methods lead to pure truth. An alternative reading, which includes more of the data available to us, makes more sense: *the closer one gets to real-world experience, the better the evidence of microdosing's substantial and lasting effects.*

†It came to be the "gold standard" after a tragedy occurred in 1961 with the release of the drug thalidomide in most countries, specifically marketed to pregnant women to prevent morning sickness. The drug caused birth defects worldwide. More than two thousand children died and ten thousand were born with shrunken or missing limbs. Although thalidomide had never been released in the United States, resulting legislation demanded far more testing before any pharmaceutical could be sold. Among the tests legislated was the double-blind. It added a huge expense to drug development, and remains so today. Its prominence came from legislation, not academic or commercial drug development scientists.

‡There is a wider problem with double-blind studies: the term itself is used in different ways by different people to mean different things. As the conclusion to one study of the term puts it, "'Double blind' and its derivatives are terms with little to recommend their continued use. Eliminating the use of adjectives that impart a false specificity to the item would reduce misinterpretations" (Lang and Stroup, 2020).

Drug effects were among the earliest areas considered by members of the Royal Society. Jay writes: "This was also the case for drugs that acted on the mind . . . the changes in thought, mood, sensation, or perception they produced were secondary qualities. . . . There was no correct or perfect way to present them, yet they offered unique insights into mental functioning."[13]

Their solution, still practiced today, can be seen in two reports described by Jay.

> Robert Hooke, curator of experiments at the Royal Society, provided some of the earliest testimony, describing in detail the effects of the many drugs he used. . . . Hooke documented impressions not just of alcohol, chocolate, tea, coffee, and tobacco, but also of cannabis. . . . Hooke detailed his own experience with the drug, in the then preferred third person:
> "This Powder . . . doth, in a short Time, quite take away the Memory & Understanding . . . being unable to speak a Word of Sense; yet is he very merry, and laughs, and sings, and speaks Words without any Coherence . . . yet is he not giddy, or drunk, but walks and dances and sheweth many odd Tricks; after a little Time, he falls asleep, and sleepeth very soundly and quietly; and when he wakes, he finds himself mightily refresh'd, and exceeding hungry."

Jay continues: "For the generation that followed, however, subjectivity was the new frontier of scientific knowledge . . . the world as received via the senses was not the accurate reflection of an external reality but a construct, shaped by the human senses and limited by the parameters of the human mind."[14]

The second historical report is from the notes of Humphry Davy, later president of the Royal Society, who at age twenty was an assistant in a medical and research institution when he discovered the effects of nitrous oxide (laughing gas).

As Jay puts it, "Humphry Davy's self-experimentation with mind-altering drugs led him to develop a 'new language of feeling.'" Jay continues:

> [He] collected the escaping gas in an air holder, from which Davy inhaled through a breathing tube. As he filled his lungs, he noticed an unexpected sensation, "a highly pleasurable thrilling in the chest and extremities." As he continued, "the objects around me became dazzling and my hearing more acute," and the sensations built toward a climax in which "the sense of muscular power became greater, and at last an irresistible propensity to action was indulged in." . . . Davey leapt violently around the laboratory, shouting for joy.[15]

Davy later gave sessions offering the gas to friends and friends of friends, requesting only a report of their experience in return.

This was then, and remains today, the natural way to study inner states—experience them and report.

The history of modern psychedelics follows this same pattern. Albert Hofmann's report on the effects of LSD, having taken what he imagined (in error) to be an extremely small dose (250 micrograms), and Aldous Huxley's still popular descriptive book of his first high-dose spiritual experience, *The Doors of Perception*, published in 1954, were culture changers. Equally important first reports came from Tim Leary and Ram Dass. The well-designed and controlled research of the 1960s—some forty thousand subjects were given LSD in diverse settings for a variety of conditions—attracted little attention; instead, it was these popular public reports that drove the popularity of psychedelics and later their repression.

Modern microdosing also began with personal reports preceding any formal research. Using the same methodology used by Hooke and Davy, Jim asked people he knew and those they knew to try microdosing. All he asked of them was their reports as to what they noticed had happened. From those reports, modern microdosing began.

The lack of psychedelic effects and the surprisingly wide range of positive health changes stood out. Many of those early results, now verified through conventional research paradigms, are scattered throughout this book.

The citizen science reports in this book are a contemporary version of the centuries-old tradition begun by the Royal Society: accumulating individual reports, looking for similarities, then extrapolating those similarities until they are considered likely properties of the substances and situation. Unfortunately, as a result of the dominance of objective evidence measurements in other areas of neuroscience, some health professionals still denigrate the value of subjective evidence.

This divide is ending as more appropriate microdosing research now focuses directly on objective correlates of subjective experiences. For example, we now have measurements of brain waves and blood flow changes to different areas of the brain that have an identical signature to those for higher doses, only at lower amplitude. Additionally, the 2024 study by Conor Murray et al. that focused on measuring "neural complexity" added more proof.* Concerns that microdosing results are based only on placebo are now dropping away as there is less dependence on self-reports as the primary source of evidence.

Given the almost wholesale acceptance of data, data analysis, and the use of large groups with averaged numerical results, it's not surprising that professionals who have only used these methods are unfamiliar with the explanatory power of explicit, detailed individual reports. Using the right tools and asking the right questions is the first step in discovering almost anything. For the subjective parts of our experience,

---

*This 2024 study showed something else that truly stood out. Test subjects who received 13 micrograms of LSD (just slightly above our average recommended range for LSD microdosing) experienced a number of measured beneficial effects that were no longer present when 26 micrograms were given. That is, it may not be so much that microdosing provides a small version of the benefits of higher doses in a less intense package spread out over time but rather that the true sweet spot for at least some beneficial effects is found only at the microdose level.

personal reports have, from the beginning, been the right tool, and will likely remain a key component of any investigative toolkit.

Citizen Science

What is "Citizen Science," who participates, and how does it work?

"Citizen Science" is a term used throughout this book as if it were commonly known. Created during the mid-1990s and defined in several ways, the term itself was added to the *Oxford English Dictionary* only in 2014. The definition is "scientific work undertaken by members of the general public, often in collaboration with or under the direction of professional scientists and scientific institutions."[16]

Its usual meaning, therefore, is about citizens working "often," but not always, with those who have been trained in very specific kinds of thinking and use of specialized tools. We are using citizen science in the older sense—a meaning that comes from before the term "scientist" was even invented—of men and women observing, recording, and sharing what they've found. Specifically, with microdosing, citizen scientists from all over the world have been observing, recording, and sharing their observations about their own feelings, behaviors, and changes in physical and emotional conditions. Most often, they have written a summary of what they felt was important and wanted others to know. It might have been called "volunteer science," since people do it of their own volition—not as a job or obligation but as a gift.

At its core, citizen science is a pay-it-forward activity where people contribute their own experiences—their concerns and difficulties, but also their surprises and successes—so that newcomers can start their own journeys with more knowledge. The goal is not just to avoid making mistakes but to not repeat those already made and noted by others.

Citizen science benefits everyone by pointing specialists in more fruitful directions. Imagine landing on an unexplored island filled with animals, plants, fungi, insects, and mineral deposits. The first discoverers would have no idea what they would find in any direction, but by making notes and maps, and sharing what they found, they would make things vastly easier for the next group landing on the island to identify what was of interest, what they needed, where the prime shelter and food spots were, and so on.

Microdosing began as that remarkable island. Nobody quite knew what was on it, what was safe, beneficial, or delightful, or what was difficult, dangerous, or debilitating.

This book is a collection of those early explorations and others still ongoing as it is being completed. It is the work of thousands of people, all of whom made a commitment so that their contributions could be of use to others.

It is likely that many of you who are reading this book will become part of this community of citizen scientists. Through observing yourself and perhaps sharing your experiences, you will pioneer new ways to apply and integrate what you've read here, along with what else is discovered going forward.

We thank you for your contributions, should you choose to participate.

Placebo Effect

My psychology professor says that microdosing just works by placebo effect and there's nothing real there. I've been microdosing for two months and stopped taking Adderall for the first time in five years. How can I answer him without being a smart-ass?

The consensus viewpoint is rapidly evolving on this question. According to neuroscientist Conor Murray, to whom we refer elsewhere:

[Recent research] certainly to me, completely puts to bed
the question of whether . . . microdoses are placebos. They're

certainly not, we have that evidence in. . . . And I think the community has just been caught up on that question because it's . . . a controversial thing to talk about. But we don't need to talk about that anymore (Murray, 2024 interview).

Placebo is Latin for *I will please* and refers to a treatment that appears real but is designed to have no therapeutic benefit. When a person's physical or mental health appears to improve after taking such an inactive placebo treatment, the "placebo effect" is said to have occurred.* What your professor is saying—he's likely just repeating what he's read in journals and popular articles—is that some microdosing studies seem to show that the only effects came from people's positive expectations. The proof: people taking the placebo (an inert sugar pill) showed the same kinds of changes as people actually taking microdoses.

We agree with those researchers who state that having a positive expectation—especially if it's based on hearing from people you know and respect that microdosing has been good for them—will likely improve your experience and even enhance the effects.

Based on our own experience and what we've heard from many people we know, we have no doubt as to the benefits of affirmations and positive expectations when using psychedelics. We see these effects most clearly in high-dose clinical studies, but to a lesser degree in microdosing as well.

Microdosing, however, clearly goes beyond just expectations and placebo: many thousands of reports and a growing number of research studies show there are undeniable effects from microdosing, some of which are apparently impervious to expectations, positive or negative.

---

*The opposite of placebo is "nocebo," where someone's negative expectations regarding an inert treatment cause a negative effect. A wonderful example is a baseball game with a dozen hot dog stands throughout the ballpark. At some point the PA system announces that people who ate at one of the hot dog stands are getting sick. This causes a dramatic rise of sudden upset stomachs and nausea throughout the ballpark among all the hot dog eaters, since everyone assumes it might have been *their* hot dog stand.

Sarah Hashkes (2022) summarizes several studies: "Research shows that 3 mg of psilocybin activated around 40% of the brain's 5ht2a receptors. As little as 5 micrograms of LSD enhanced sustained attention and improved positive mood and 10 micrograms increased subjective reports of 'good drug effect.'"[17]

Dustin Marlan (2022) describes additional studies: "Researchers have shown changes in brain conductivity and activity through neuroimaging technology after a single low dose of LSD similar to those seen with larger doses. . . . Another study too found that microdosing psilocybin had similar effects on the brain as compared to a macrodose of the substance." And in 2024, a study by Conor Murray (Murray et al., 2024) showed, as Grace Wade put it, that "microdosing LSD increases the complexity of your brain signals" as "a measure of consciousness called neural complexity increases even with small doses of LSD."[18]

Early on, there was considerable interest in demonstrating the nonactivity of microdosing, but now most research is moving closer to naturalistic settings that are more representative of real-world microdosing use. Vince Polito, best known for his review of microdosing studies showing limited, if any, changes, points out the inherent limitations of even the best studies and concludes, "I suggest that it is premature to rule out a pharmacological effect of microdosing."[19] One of the limitations he sees is "all lab-based studies to date have investigated healthy populations. It may be there are clinical benefits specific to particular conditions. Microdosers regularly report considerable positive impacts from microdosing. As a striking example, in one study, more than 50% of respondents reported ceasing traditional medications after they started microdosing."[20]

As with any health-enhancing substance, different individuals in different situations will experience differing effects. For some people, changes in their own expectations may be the only effect. However, at least in the populations that we have access to, *reported and perceived changes in enhanced capacities and health conditions far exceed the possibility of just being explained by placebo and expectation effects.* We're back to observational science, square one.

The bottom line, though, is that daily questionnaires showed very credible evidence of improved ratings of creativity, connectedness, energy, [and] happiness, relative to placebo. Microdoses are not a placebo effect.
—Conor Murray (Murray, 2024 training video)

Expectancy

Professor Nutt says that expectations cause the actual effect when people take microdoses, not the psychedelic. What gives?

We apologize for giving a more technical answer than we might prefer, but as this is a controversy among researchers, we will quote the earlier research that frames this issue, as well as the later research that apparently resolves it.

We have already quoted Dr. Nutt more than once because of his objectivity and candor in reporting experimental findings. This was his position in 2023 on the role of expectations in predicting microdosing effects:

> At Imperial College we wanted to find out more about the impact of expectations on microdosing. The team surveyed people before they began their own microdosing regimen, to ask them what they thought they'd get from it. After four weeks of their regimen, they surveyed them again. People reported that microdosing had improved their well-being, mood and performance. They said it reduced symptoms of anxiety and depression and increased resilience, social connections, agreeableness and psychological flexibility. . . .
>
> However, there was a kicker: the subjects' positive expectations predicted their positive effects, suggesting a significant placebo response at work. . . . Our conclusion? Microdosing does work . . . but people's beliefs about it are more important than the drug itself.[21]

However, this conclusion was questioned by a later double-blind LSD study done in New Zealand* (Allen et al., 2023). Lasting six weeks, its subjects were healthy males with no prior microdosing experience, and it made use of the Fadiman protocol, a wearable sleep monitor, and a daily check-in. Conor Murray, while discussing this study on a live audio chat in the Flourish Academy on the Clubhouse app in April 2024, focused briefly on the expectations data, noting results that did not support Nutt's conclusion:

> On the microdose days [the subjects] had increased creativity, increased connectedness to others, and positive mood. And when you looked at that, compared to their expectations of what would happen, it was significantly different. . . .
> That was really compelling evidence . . . that on microdose days, these healthy folks have these very meaningful changes.[22]

Additionally, a carefully designed study in Colombia (Suarez et al., 2023) included 105 individuals microdosing psilocybin, nineteen of whom completed logs over the full forty days. (Fadiman protocol, including several weeks off.) The study was undertaken to discover and determine the numerous reported effects of microdosing variables, including recording the difference between initial expectations and eventual results.

> Respondents generally obtained more benefits than they initially expected. On average respondents achieved 0.7 more benefits than they sought [on a scale of -2 to +4]. In addition, 42% of respondents received one or more of the expected benefits. Only 25% of the participants did not obtain sufficient benefits in relation to their initial motivations.
> This is one of the most relevant findings. . . . One of

---

*This study was widely described in popular media because one effect that was discovered was that participants slept significantly longer the second day after a microdose. This was a novel and unexpected result.

the main debates in current microdosing research revolves around whether the positive effects achieved by microdosers are explained by the positive expectations about the results of the practice (Szigeti, 2021). The findings presented here are consistent with some of the studies where microdosers tend to obtain broader benefits than those sought (Polio and Stevenson, 2019) . . . the findings . . . indicate that the practice of microdosing ended up generating benefits in aspects that were not part of the initial motivations of the microdosers.

This diagram, redrawn from the published article and translated into English, makes it easy to see that most of the benefits reported were unanticipated.

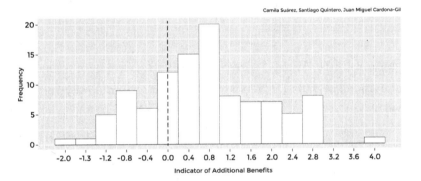

Camila Suárez, Santiago Quintero, Juan Miguel Cardona-Gil

Distribution of additional benefits to those expected. The indicated frequency of additional benefits is presented. The values to the right of the dotted mark above 0 indicate people with a higher number of benefits than expected (according to the motivations used to initiate microdosing).

The chart shows that most people had more positive results than they anticipated or expected,
Each rectangle shows (graphically) the number of people with different expectation scores.
If expectations were the only variable and were totally predictive, all subjects would be on the dotted central line.

The odds of these kinds of results happening by chance are quite small. Taken together with the New Zealand study, we can say that while some early researchers were concerned that microdosing's reported effects were only or primarily due to a combination of placebo and expectation effects, we can now put those speculations to rest. We have covered the issues about placebo elsewhere; here we let the reported research results about expectations end this controversy.

Neuroplasticity, Neurogenesis, and the Default Mode Network

I keep hearing these terms. What do they mean, and what do I need to know about them?

These concepts attract a great deal of scientific and media attention, and will continue to do so for the foreseeable future. Let's start with PositivePsychology.com's definitions of the first two:

> Although related, neuroplasticity and neurogenesis are two different concepts. Neuroplasticity is the ability of the brain to form new connections and pathways and change how its circuits are wired; neurogenesis is the . . . ability of the brain to grow new neurons.[23]

Neurogenesis, which is relatively rare and appears to be of secondary importance, refers to the birth or creation of *new* neurons, while neuroplasticity refers to how the brain adapts to experience.

Neuroplasticity physically alters existing neurons as well as changes, reorganizes, and assembles and reassembles ("rewires") networks of neurons that communicate with each other. "Neuroplasticity denotes the nervous system's ability to reorganize its structure and function and adapt to its dynamic environment. Throughout the lifespan, neuroplasticity is essential for learning, memory, and recovery from neurological insults, as well as adapting to life experience."[24]

The term "plasticity"* was first used in *The Principles of Psychology* (1890) by the psychologist and philosopher William James. James's focus was on "how learning, skill acquisition, interpersonal and social

---

*The first fully synthetic plastic was made in 1907, but the use of natural plastics—including animal horn (pliable when heated), amber, and rubber—goes back to antiquity. The 1860s saw the invention of the first plastics manufactured from natural materials, at which point "plastic"—from the Greek "plastikos," meaning to form or mold—began to be used as a noun.

influences . . . can influence . . . the physical structure of the brain, modifying and establishing new relationships and neural circuits."[25] James wrote:

> Plasticity . . . means the possession of a structure weak enough to yield to an influence, but strong enough not to yield all at once. Each relatively stable phase of equilibrium in such a structure is marked by what we may call a new set of habits. Organic matter, especially nervous tissues, seem to be endowed with a very extraordinary degree of plasticity of this sort.[26]

Neuroplasticity makes it possible for new combinations of neurons and new networks of neurons to signal and connect with each other, enabling different parts of the body, brain, and mind to communicate. It can be useful to think of neuroplasticity as our ability to learn and lock in new behaviors and patterns that serve us . . . and let go of ones that don't. Note that while increased neuroplasticity is often assumed to be beneficial, that's not always the case.

To understand how neuroplasticity works, let's begin with a brief review of the nature of neurons. Neurons are specialized cells in animal and human bodies that transmit information throughout the body's nervous system using electrochemical signals and other means of communication. ("Neurons engage in multiple types of communication simultaneously,"[27] which includes the use of neurotransmitters, electrical signals, and synchronizing brain waves.) As the cells that send messages through the body, neurons enable us to feel, move, eat, think . . . and do almost everything else.

Key structural and functional elements of neurons include:

- **Nucleus:** Located in the neuron's main body, it contains DNA and is the control center.
- **Dendrites:** Small branches that reach out and pick up signals from other neurons.

- **Axon:** A long thin wire-like part stretching out from the neuron to send signals to other neurons.
- **Myelin Sheath:** An insulating coating on axons that speeds signals along.
- **Axon Terminals:** Found at the end of the axon, they send signals to the next neuron.
- **Synapses:** The tiny gaps between neurons where signals are passed.

Currently, it's believed that the human body contains about 135 billion neurons. Roughly 120 billion are in the central nervous system (CNS) in the brain and spine, with another 15 billion or so in the peripheral nervous system. These include *afferent neurons* carrying sensory information from the outside world to our brain and *efferent neurons* carrying motor or action initiating information from the CNS to the body's muscles and glands. Additionally, there are up to 600 million neurons in the *enteric nervous system* governing the functions of the gastrointestinal tract.

The vast majority of neuroplasticity research focuses on the CNS, particularly the brain. However, considering the wide range of effects attributed to macrodosing and microdosing, it's likely some of the important actions are going on *outside* the brain. Not only are more than 10 percent of our neurons in places other than the brain, but anyone who's had an upset stomach affect their mood has a sense of the importance of "the brain in the gut."

Neurons have a companion, *glial cells.* There are roughly the same number of glial cells in the CNS as there are neurons, with the three main types being *astrocytes, oligodendrocytes,* and *microglia.* While glial cells used to be thought of as mainly unimportant and uninteresting "helper" cells, scientific opinion has been shifting over time. (Why would the brain and spine contain a hundred billion of something that didn't really do anything?) According to Dzyubenko and Hermann (2023), glial cells have multiple direct effects on neuroplasticity.

Emerging evidence indicates that glial cells actively shape neuroplasticity, allowing for highly flexible regulation of synaptic transmission, neuronal excitability, and network synchronization. Astrocytes regulate synaptogenesis, stabilize synaptic connectivity, and preserve the balance between excitation and inhibition in neuronal networks. Microglia . . . continuously monitor and sculpt synapse, allowing for the remodeling of brain circuits.[28]

An earlier paper (Kargbo, 2003) stated, "It is apparent that psychedelics activate ensembles of excitatory neurons, inhibitory interneurons, and non-neuronal cells like astrocytes and glia as well as increase synaptic density and connections between neurons."[29] The mention of astrocytes is significant, as astrocytes contain 5-HT(2A) or serotonin receptors, which are particularly relevant to theories as to which types of cells are affected by classic psychedelics.* However, there has been relatively little focus on the role of glial cells in augmenting or modulating neuroplasticity.

The Science: Now let's turn to the actual science. We'll give you the rough contours: the outlines of what neuroscientists have been doing so far, where their studies are pointing, and what we can expect in the future.

One area of agreement is that the great majority of the theoretical and experimental focus should rightly remain on neuroplasticity and *not* neurogenesis. While it is sometimes thought that the adult human brain creates new neurons, especially in the hippocampus—although at a much lesser rate than in newborns and children—it is by no means settled science.

---

*A large percentage of psychedelic research has focused on the function, regulation, and effect of a single receptor—the 5-HT(2A) receptor. However, other neuroreceptors also play important roles with the biochemistry of psychedelics, including the 5-HT(2C) receptor, the mGlu2 receptor (a glutamate receptor), D2 receptors, which interact with dopamine, sigma receptors, and other glutamate receptors like AMPA and NMDA. We wouldn't be surprised if over time the focus on the 5-HT(2A) receptor diminishes as the role of other receptors becomes clearer.

Neuroscientist and educator Andrew Huberman, while noting that there is some evidence for neurogenesis in adult human brains in the dentate gyrus and other areas of the hippocampus, emphasizes that neurogenesis is going to be a very minor factor when it comes to psychedelic neuroplasticity:

> Neurogenesis is not a prominent feature of learning and
> acquisition of new skills, new ideas, or new emotional states
> [and] is not really the dominant mode of changing neural
> circuitry in adult humans. It might be a player in adolescence,
> in young childhood. It is certainly a player before we are born,
> when we are still in utero. . . . While neurogenesis is a really
> sticky idea, and it makes great headlines, the addition of new
> neurons is not really the way that the brain changes under
> psilocybin, other psychedelics, or just generally. It's perhaps
> responsible for maybe 1 to 2%—and I'm being generous
> there—of the rewiring events that are going to be most im-
> portant for all of us.[30]

Putting neurogenesis aside, we can turn to the two main types of neuroplasticity research. The first focuses on rats and mice—and occasionally primates—who are given psychedelics and then compared with similar mice and rats exposed to the same conditions and stimuli, but not given psychedelics. A recent paper notes that a central problem in psychedelic research is that we measure very different things in animals than we measure in humans. And that while it's a common assumption that what's true in mice *should* be true in humans, this is no more than an assumption, and in many cases has been proven wrong (Heifets and Olson, 2023).

As the key 2023 neuroplasticity paper by Calder and Hasler demonstrates,[31] this type of research has shown a variety of physical results in rodents given psychedelics (often just a single high dose):

- Increases in density of synapses, dendrites, and dendritic spines.
- Increases in rates of dendritogenesis (growth of new dendrites), synaptogenesis (new synapses), and spinogenesis (new dendrite spines).
- Increased BDNF protein (brain-derived neurotrophic factor, a protein found in the brain and spinal cord that is essential to neural development and health).
- Moliner et al. (2023) have shown that with powerful affinity, "[LSD] and psilocybin directly bind to Trkb," the neuroreceptor for BDNF.[32]
- Upregulation (or increased production of) plasticity-related genes.
- Upregulation of BDNF messenger RNA.
- Upregulation of IEGs (immediately early genes), which are associated with synaptic plasticity and synaptogenesis.

From these rodent studies we know that there are actual physical and functional changes made to neurons at the DNA expression level, as well as physical and functional observable changes that make it easier for them to connect to other neurons. According to Calder and Hasler, "Significant progress has been made toward understanding how psychedelics affect neuroplasticity. Data thus far supports the theory that psychedelics stimulate dendritogenesis, synaptogenesis, and the upregulation of plasticity-related genes . . . affecting the cortex in particular."[33]

In distinction to rodent-based studies, human-based studies primarily make use of:

- Functional MRI (magnetic resonance imaging) and PET (positron emission tomography) scans showing that psychedelics alter brain connectivity and blood flow patterns.
- Electrophysiology studies conducted using an EEG (electroencephalogram) or MEG (magnetoencephalography), showing

changed oscillatory activity (speed of firing) and synchronization in the brain.

- Ultrasound studies revealing patterns of blood flow and measuring changes in the structure and connectivity of brain networks.
- Blood plasma samples showing circulating BDNF levels in human volunteers.
- Survey questionnaire studies relating to participants' perceived experiences taking different doses of different substances (sometimes with a placebo control).

Brain and ultrasound scans are also used with live rodents to measure changes in blood flow, oscillatory activity, synchronization, and so on.

Human-based studies have looked at whether lower doses, including microdoses, produce neuroplasticity in a similar manner to higher doses, even if at a proportionately reduced volume or impact level. The work of the neurologist Evan Lewis, referring to both brain scans and BDNF plasma levels, speaks to this: "We have concrete, laboratory-based evidence that the serotonergic psychedelics—like psilocybin, DMT, ayahuasca, and LSD—show markers of neuroplasticity that seem to vary with dose amount and how frequently the dose is administered."[34] Similarly, Hirschfeld et al. (2023) state:

> LSD doses below 10 µg [micrograms] or 20 µg have previously been proposed as the "microdosing" range of LSD. The fitted curves in our analysis show an onset of effects below 20 µg LSD base. For instance, visual phenomena . . . show an x-axis intercept at around 10 µg, and at 20 µg reach around 10% of the maximum score. These effects are unlikely due to placebo effects. . . . Most studies below 20 µg . . . make the microdosing range of 0–20 µg plausible.[35]

There appears, then, to be a dose-response curve extending down into the microdose range, so that people who take microdoses will be experiencing real physiological effects, including those associated with neuroplasticity.

More skeptical scientists point to mixed results. According to Calder and Hasler:

> Though these studies suggest that psychedelics probably pro-
> mote neuroplasticity in a dose-dependent manner, clear dose-
> response effects on neuroplasticity have not been established
> in humans. Sub-hallucinogenic doses of between 5 and 20 µg
> LSD produced significant short-term enhancements in plasma
> BDNF. However, a similar study using doses of between 25 µg
> and 200 µg LSD only found significant effects on BDNF at
> 200 µg, and another failed to find significant changes even at
> this dose. Perhaps using different methods, future research
> should seek to clarify the minimum and optimal doses for
> stimulating neuroplasticity with different psychedelics.[36]

Moving beyond these questions, it may be more useful to inquire as to the importance and significance of new combinations of neurons and new networks of neurons signaling each other, enabling different parts of the body, brain, and mind to communicate. By facilitating neuroplasticity at the cellular and network levels, psychedelics create an opportunity to change patterns in brain activity and behavior. We can—with proper planning, intention, and focus—bio-physiologically rewire our brains to create, instantiate, and propagate more desirable ways of being . . . and let go of undesirable ones.

Creating new (and letting go of old) patterns is facilitated by different networks of neurons—and thereby different parts of the brain, body, and mind—connecting with each other. Andrew Huberman notes that what we are interested in is "enhanced lateral connectivity, less hierarchical organization, [and] effectively more interconnection and communication between different brain areas."[37] He emphasizes the importance of *pyramidal* neurons (named for their pyramid-like shape), which seem particularly good at forming new structures capable of sending signals to areas of the brain that would otherwise not be reached. As one study states, "through their primary glutamate or serotonin receptor targets, ketamine and psychedelics [psilocybin, lysergic acid diethylamide (LSD), and N,N-dimethyltryptamine (DMT)] induce synaptic, structural, and functional changes, particularly in pyramidal neurons in the prefrontal cortex."[38]

More Neuroplasticity *Isn't* Always Better

> Just because something invokes neuroplasticity...
> does not mean that it is necessarily therapeutic.
> For neuroplasticity to be therapeutic, it has to
> be adaptive, it has to allow someone to function
> better in life than they did previously.
> —Andrew Huberman, neuroscientist and educator

Increased neuroplasticity is often automatically considered a good thing, but sometimes it isn't. For example, some types of neuroplasticity—such as what amphetamines and cocaine produce—are generally not considered beneficial or desirable. And if you find yourself in a strongly neuroplastic condition (suppose you've taken a macrodose) and are experiencing emotional, physical, or other difficulties, your "plastic" mind-state may imprint trauma or negativity, or leave you stuck in a part of you that does something crazy or dangerous. (Yes, like the seriously depressed off-duty pilot who took a macrodose of mushrooms in 2023 and forty-eight hours later tried to end a nightmarish multiday "dream" he was having by bringing down an airplane full of people. Fortunately, he did not succeed.)

As *The Atlantic* author Richard A. Friedman put it in a 2023 article, "all those changes aren't necessarily all *good*. Neuroplasticity just means that your brain—and your mind—is put into a state where it is more easily influenced. The effect is a bit like putting a glass vase back into the kiln, which makes it pliable and easy to reshape. Of course you can make the vase more functional and beautiful, but you might also turn it into a mess."[39]

What's important is whether the neuroplasticity you experience allows you to learn and encode new thoughts, feelings, and behaviors, or enables you to let go of dysfunctional memories, pain, and behavioral patterns. Not enough neuroplasticity throws up roadblocks as to what you're capable of learning, doing, and accomplishing, but too much neuroplasticity at the wrong time can result in substantial challenges and difficulties.

Default Mode Network (DMN)

Especially with regard to letting go of dysfunctional patterns, there has been a great deal of research and speculation as to how psychedelics disrupt and suspend the normal activity of what is called the default mode network or DMN. This set of interconnected brain regions is active when we're awake and at rest but have no particular focus, and is associated with self-reflection, wandering thoughts, and daydreaming.

When our DMN is turned down or off, it becomes easier for parts of our brain, body, and mind to connect with each other in new and more functional ways.* On a physical level, this may enable the reconnection of neural pathways to injured or aging parts of the body, or might enable the part of you that's in love with life to "speak to"—communicate with—another part of you that is unhappy or depressed. Similarly, if you have a chronic pain condition or circuit in your brain that is easily triggered into withdrawal, rage, or fear, you may find it easier than usual

---

*More connectivity generally—and the suspension and turning down of our brain's and mind's normal ways of being—has also been described in terms of an "entropic effect." The thought here is that psychedelics (including microdoses) create—or stop the suppression of—the degree of entropy characteristic of normal consciousness, resulting in new patterns of connection in the brain on the neural and network levels. This concept has been seemingly confirmed by J. Siegel et al.'s widely reported 2024 study, "Psilocybin Desynchronizes the Human Brain." A related idea is "metaplasticity," referring to the "plasticity of neuroplasticity." The focus here is on how biochemical and physiological changes in neurons affect their overall ability to generate even more plasticity (e.g., how the previous activity at a synapse affects current and future activity).

to release that pain circuit—that particular mental or psychophysiological reflex.

A key pragmatic question is **how long does neuroplasticity last?** This is scientifically discussed in terms of "open periods," "critical periods," and "windows" of neuroplasticity. "Open periods" are times when the brain is especially open, imprintable, and sensitive to environmental input. "Critical periods" refer to specific times during childhood and adolescence when the brain undergoes rapid development and rewiring while powerfully purging unwanted connections. Finally, there are "windows of neuroplasticity," referring to specific time periods when the brain is more plastic than normal, meaning more capable of forming new connections and breaking old ones.

Based both on animal and human research, neuroplasticity markers or direct measurements last longer than the amount of time the psychedelic substance has its greatest real-time subjective impact, that is, in the first several hours after ingestion. Calder and Hasler write:

> Though neuroplasticity may increase within several hours, the peak effects may come later. . . . Enhanced neuroplasticity may also last for several days. . . . In humans, research has uncovered changes in brain function which lasted at least 1 month after treatment with psilocybin. . . . These data suggest that various signs of enhanced neuroplasticity arise within 1–6 hours, with changes in gene expression appearing earliest and changes in cell morphology and synapse organization arising later. The increased rate of dendritogenesis may taper off within 5 days, however, neuroplastic changes which arise during this period of neuronal growth may last for at least 1 month.[40]

These findings are consistent with what we know from individual reports. The "afterglow," where one is still affected after a large-dose experience, has long been part of psychedelic lore. That is, for a number of days afterward, people feel—and are experienced by others as being—

noticeably different, even "lit up" or "turned on" in a distinct way. In microdosing, the second-day effect is similar, but scaled down.

In his podcast episode "How Psilocybin Can Rewire Our Brain," Andrew Huberman sheds light on neuroplasticity windows:

> The best way to think about psilocybin and other psychedelics is that they initiate the neuroplasticity process, but they are *not* the neuroplasticity process itself, and the [psychedelic] journey itself is not where all the neuroplasticity occurs. We know that for sure. . . . Think of them [psychedelics] as a *wedge* that gets underneath the boulder that is the neuroplasticity that gets rolling forward. And then think about whether or not the plasticity is adaptive or maladaptive, whether or not it actually serves you in your life on a daily basis or not, depending on whether or not you are using your conscious brain to move that boulder in a particular direction . . . not just bulldozing through things and destroying them but clearing a path through old ineffective, maybe even destructive, patterns of thoughts or emotions.[41]

We could say that microdosing puts a series of micro-wedges under our neuroplasticity boulders, cumulatively giving us the ability and opportunity to make changes.

As for what you *need* to know and how to best take advantage of everything we've covered here, there are two ways to think about all this. On the one hand, *you really don't need to know anything in particular about neuroplasticity for microdosing to work well for you.* That is, if you don't understand what science knows up to this point about neuroplasticity, it will not change your experience. So, while neuroplasticity likely explains a significant part of microdosing's reported benefits, it's not really necessary to understand it scientifically.

On the other hand, understanding neuroplasticity windows may help you plan which protocol to use and how to adapt it to your own circumstances. In our discussion of ADHD, for example, we consider a protocol starting in the early evening, thereby taking advantage of the next day's neuroplasticity window. And understanding the second-day effect and being aware of reports of better sleep on the second day can help with more effective protocol and schedule planning.

It's clear that neuroplasticity won't explain *everything* about psychedelics generally or microdosing in particular. For example, the reason why psychedelics generally reduce inflammation may be related to neuroplasticity, but there's also evidence that pro-inflammatory cytokines (small proteins important in cell signaling) are directly reduced by psychedelics, yielding general anti-inflammatory effects. Similarly, the body's general return to homeostasis and the release of what we sometimes like to think of as "natural healing factors" may not specifically involve neuroplasticity. Regardless of its immediate practical value, we expect continued focus on neuroplasticity's central role in the short- and long-term future as the current psychedelic revival continues.

Inflammation

I've heard that microdosing helps reduce inflammation. Is that really true, and if so, how much do we know about it?

During the several years it took to write this book, there has been considerable progress in understanding the physiological underpinnings that explain some of the prominent effects of psychedelics. At the same time, the renewed interest in, availability of, and commercial possibilities for research and general use have led to an exponential increase in the amount of attention psychedelics receive in the media. A small study may be followed by a herd of articles in the popular press only to later be refuted by another article with little or no press attention.

Very little of the science focuses on real-life experience. As our primary focus has been on detailed individual reports, it has made us cautious in assuming that the popular narrative or the peer-reviewed scientific journal narrative is definitive.

In looking at inflammation—perhaps one of the most important purely physiological processes affected by different psychedelics—much of the science has been tentative, and so too was our initial description. Rather than simply describe our current position, we'll begin with our initial tentative understanding and tentative language—both of which fall away with the coming of definitive research—so you can see where we are today with the same eyes that we do.

I've heard that microdosing reduces inflammation. Is that why people say their whole body feels better?

[Our initial answer] Inflammation is "the process by which the immune system recognizes and removes harmful and foreign stimuli and begins the healing process. [It] can be either acute or chronic."[42] Many illnesses and conditions can cause inflammation, resulting in redness, swelling, rash, warmth, pain, and loss of function. As a built-in bodily response to protect us from infections, injuries, and autoimmune problems, inflammation is a response to something that has stressed the body.

However, *inflammation can also cause or lead to certain diseases,* especially when it is persistent and contributes to a wide range of conditions, from heart disease, cancer, and diabetes to arthritis and bowel disease. Autoimmune diseases, where inflammation results from the body's immune system mistakenly attacking healthy tissue, are often difficult to treat. Finally, "as we grow older, aches and pains can become a chronic way of life" as there is "an uptick in inflammatory molecules over the course of a lifetime. . . . The link between age, inflammation, and disease is so well established, it has a name: inflammaging."[43]

It has long been thought that psychedelics have an anti-inflammatory effect. Early scientific evidence was promising along multiple fronts, with several plausible physiological explanatory mechanisms under active research in animal and human studies. These included anti-inflammatory effects directly modulated by the 5-HT(2A) receptor. There was also increasing interest in the ability of psychedelics to mediate cytokines—small proteins that are crucial in cell signaling—suppressing pro-inflammatory ones and encouraging anti-inflammatory ones. The connection between psychedelics, the gut biome (see the earlier discussion of inflammatory bowel disease), and inflammation is also actively studied. Changes in neuroplasticity are often linked to discussions on why psychedelics may reduce inflammation.

An increasing amount of animal and human research is happening along these fronts, including markers of reduced inflammation in human blood, with almost all of it being high-dose research. The upshot of these studies is that they "have confirmed the capacity of psychedelics to modulate processes that perpetuate chronic low-grade inflammation and thus exert significant therapeutic effects in a diverse array of preclinical disease models, including asthma, atherosclerosis, inflammatory bowel disease, and retinal disease."[44]

Notwithstanding the exploration of these research vectors, at this point, the science of inflammation and psychedelics generally—and microdosing in particular—is significantly less fully developed than, for example, the science of neuroplasticity. All one study managed to conclude is that "while the area of research is quite underdeveloped, there is some evidence that psychedelic compounds have anti-inflammatory and immune-modulating systems."[45]

We think there is more than just "some evidence"—published research cited elsewhere in this book, as well as considerable real-world evidence—to support the conclusion that psychedelics have anti-inflammatory properties.

Acknowledging that the confirmatory science we now have is less developed than it one day will be, let's return to the real-world evidence. Four examples of many conditions where inflammation plays a key role are described in detail earlier:

- asthma
- Ehlers-Danlos syndrome

- inflammatory bowel disease
- long COVID

Finally, the most common real-world report we've heard about microdosing is that it *tends to make people feel better*. While that can be for many reasons, a reduction of inflammation seems likely to be one.

Inflammation may be reduced by interventions such as dietary changes, stress management techniques, meditation, breathing exercises, adequate sleep, cold therapy, and so on. As research and real-world evidence continue to accumulate, the effects of microdosing in treating inflammation will be better understood. From what we know already, it may soon become part of conventional anti-inflammatory therapeutic approaches and protocols.

[Our more recent answer] **Settled Science**: A 2022 article by Charles Nichols, "Anti-inflammatory Therapeutics,"[46] makes clear that prior speculations were correct: *there is now definitive data about the effectiveness of psychedelics in reducing inflammation.*

After pointing out that virtually all psychedelic research and the way they work has focused on brain and consciousness changes, Nichols states, "Remarkably, we have discovered that psychedelics are also *potent anti-inflammatories and immunomodulators* in peripheral tissues."[47] (Emphasis added.) The paper reviews what is known about this, considers "the development of psychedelics as potential therapeutics for human inflammatory disease," and explains why "certain psychedelics represent a new class of . . . small molecule, highly bioavailable, anti-inflammatory that is steroid sparing and efficacious at sub-behavioral levels,"[48] and which can be used potentially for treatment and prevention of many diseases and conditions with an inflammatory component.

Potential Heart Damage Concerns

I've read that taking microdoses over long periods of time can lead to heart damage. Scary! Is it true?

A letter to the Harvard Law School "Bill of Health" blog from a pharmacy professor strongly states this concern:

> There is compelling theoretical evidence to suggest prolonged and repeated microdosing may cause valvular heart disease (VHD).[49]

We corresponded with him to learn more about what he meant by "theoretical" and "suggest." He pointed to a study of twenty-nine high-use MDMA users (an average of 3.6 tablets or doses per week over 6.1 years). In that study, 28 percent of those people developed symptoms of VHD.[50] While MDMA is not a true psychedelic, it does appear to affect some of the same neurons as psychedelics. However, if you have any MDMA experience, you will recognize that those studied here were taking far more than anyone has ever suggested makes any sense.

The pharmacy professor acknowledged that those who microdosed— taking days off between doses and several weeks off every few months— were unlikely to be in any danger. Others who have put forth similar concerns have pointed to a diet drug that was on the market some years ago; once again, taking a daily dose many times greater than a microdose caused that heart condition. The drug was then withdrawn from the market.

The theoretical danger here is that since (a) the heart can be damaged by taking drugs that affect specific neurons, and (b) psychedelics affect those same neurons, then (c), maybe even much smaller doses spaced out over time would have the same effect.

By definition, we know that "overdosing" almost anything causes problems. Throughout this book we have highlighted the "negative effects" of taking microdoses and offered appropriate cautions. During the peak of the rave scene—from the late 1980s through the 1990s— with all-night dance parties fueled by MDMA, deaths were typically attributed in the media to the drug itself and its effects. However, careful examination has shown that most of these deaths were due to overexertion and overheating or either drinking not enough water or too much water without electrolytes (leading to fatally low blood sodium levels).[51] Taking MDMA was rarely the cause of death of the raver; not properly preparing for and addressing predictable well-known stressors was.

Most recently, a paper published in the *Journal of Psychopharmacology* surveyed the risks of microdosing with psychedelics as well as the risks associated with similar substances. It states that "some medications exhibiting a close chemical resemblance to psychedelics have been associated with the development of cardiac fibrosis and valvulopathy."[52] The authors present a table of twelve substances, including LSD, psilocybin, and psilocin, with possible links to the two conditions. Some substances were associated with these conditions, some were not.

Three substances had no information: LSD, psilocybin, and psilocin. Eighty-six peer-reviewed journal references, *but no cases, evidence, or data for any of these three.* Their conclusion was that "though the risk of fibrosis and VHD is uncertain at this point, it is important to investigate potential adverse effects seriously as microdosing gains in popularity."

We can only add that, to date, from our own and other investigators' files of microdosing individuals, we have no evidence either.

Given the burden and expense, the likelihood is low that studies measuring the long-term cardiac health of microdosers will be undertaken. Still, we agree with the general conclusion that it is important to be aware of possible dangers, even if this one will likely remain "theoretical" and "suggested."

Homeopathy and Microdosing

Is homeopathy similar to microdosing?

Widely used (especially outside the United States), *homeopathy has very little in common with microdosing.* While homeopathy and microdosing may seem similar in that they both make use of a tiny amount of active substance, they differ in substantial ways. First, microdosing rebalances or improves the functioning of many different body systems, while homeopathy is symptom-specific (and person-specific). Second, homeopathy makes use of thousands of different remedies, as opposed to the relatively few substances used for microdosing. Third, while homeopathy was created about two hundred years ago, microdosing goes back much further in human history in indigenous societies worldwide. Homeopathy is based on three assumptions:

- "Like cures like"—a condition can be cured by very small amounts of a substance that produces similar symptoms in healthy people.
- "Law of minimum dose"—the lower the dose (the more rounds of dilution and "succussion" or vigorous shaking), the greater its effectiveness. The most powerful homeopathic treatments statistically may contain less than one molecule of the original substance, while there are more than ten quadrillion molecules of LSD in a typical microdose!
- "Individualization"—a practicing homeopath conducts an in-depth interview with a new patient and individually tailors treatments for each person; it's common for two people with similar conditions to receive different treatments.

Originally created by the German physician Samuel Hahnemann (1755–1843), homeopathy is accepted as an alternative medical system in Europe—it is practiced in forty out of forty-two European nations[53] and in India. According to the US National Institutes of Health, more than two hundred million people use homeopathy regularly world-wide.[54] There is also widespread use with animals and livestock.[55] It was estimated in 2002 that in the US the number of patients using homeopathic remedies had risen fivefold in the previous seven years.[56] Homeopathy, however, is generally shunned by mainstream American medicine because of its radically different fundamental assumptions, diagnostic methods, and treatments, along with the remarkable diversity of its remedies.

Synthesized Psilocybin vs. Psychedelic Mushroom Extract

Is there any noticeable difference between synthesized and real psilocybin mushrooms?

The very short answer is "yes," they are different, and whole mushrooms are more effective. The long answer includes some background and recent research.

The reality is that the Pharmaceutical/Food and Drug Complex prefers single-substance drugs. They're easier to manufacture, measure, test, store, ship, and compare with other single-substance drugs. Nature prefers complicated mixtures of substances within a single plant or fungus.

There are more than two hundred different mushrooms containing psilocybin and a mixture of other psycho-chemicals, as well as a growing number of variations ("cultivars") from several species created by mycological investigators and explorers.

Although the difference between synthetic and full-spectrum psilocybin is an obvious question, until recently there was no research from either side. There was no benefit to the pharmaceutical companies in exploring advantages or disadvantages of the entourage substances since they had no commercial likelihood of being accepted. Meanwhile, the growing number of individual growers creating new subspecies had no access to or interest in synthetic psilocybin.

A study in Israel published in early 2024 measured the differences between using synthetic psilocybin and the mushroom extract in adult male mice. "All experiments were conducted with the investigator blind to treatment assignment" (Shahar, 2024). Measurements at three days after showed minimal increase in synaptic proteins for both conditions. However, after eleven days, the mushroom extract showed increases in a number of brain areas that the synthetics did not. "Mushroom extract demonstrated a stronger and more prolonged impact on synaptic plasticity, potentially offering unique therapeutic benefits" (NeuroScience, 2024).

The senior researchers and the psychiatrist guiding the study state that "the mushroom extract containing psilocybin may exhibit superior efficacy when compared to chemically synthesized psilocybin" (Neuro-Science, 2024).

Restated with less professional jargon, the extract showed enhanced neuroplasticity, determined to be one of the most important factors in the general healing of microdosing across multiple conditions.

This finding, that the whole mushroom "exhibits superior efficacy," confirms a widely accepted belief in the mycological and microdosing communities. However, it calls into question a great deal of the research done with synthetic psilocybin, limiting its conclusions and its results—and now and again, its lack of results—which are valid only for synthetics.

The pharmacological research, academic, and commercial worlds will likely continue to use—if only for commercial reasons and research convenience—single-substance and predominantly synthesized psychedelics. Microdosing communities worldwide will continue to have access to full-spectrum mushrooms or extracts.

In this area, the first-level question of "are there any differences?" has now been definitively answered. Second-level questions, including "In what ways do these differences affect practical issues in health and treatment?" will become more prominent as both synthetic and full-spectrum psilocybin become more legally available. The first of these studies is already underway at UCLA, measuring the difference between the two types of psilocybin on the lifespan and other variables of simpler short-lived species. Eventually separate markets will be established for each, resembling the current differences between organic and chemically treated fruits and vegetables. The difference being that, in this case, the natural version will probably be far less expensive.

Indigenous Use

As we know, indigenous people used psychedelic plants and fungi for centuries—perhaps for thousands of years—before the West did. Are you now further perpetrating the cultural appropriation and exploitation suffered by these groups?

This is a frequent charge made against companies and researchers attempting to profit from using different psychedelics as medications and is, in many cases, a realistic one.

We have strong views on this. We feel that indigenous people, certainly in the Americas, have not merely been colonized and exploited but were subject to the worst human carnage in history—a centuries-long genocide of imported plagues and barbarous atrocities that annihilated 95 percent of their populations.[57] The driving forces here were a desire for profit supported by a Christian theology that reduced non-Christians to little more than objects.

> **It can never be forgotten or forgiven, and the destruction can never be rectified.**

We are looking forward to living in a world in which such things never happen again.

A welcome first step in this direction recently took place when "an

Indigenous-led globally represented group of practitioners, activists, scholars, lawyers, and human rights defenders came together with the purpose of formulating a set of ethical guidelines concerning traditional Indigenous medicines [in] current use in Western psychedelic research and practice."[58] The eight ethical principles set forth by Yuria Celidwen, Nicole Redvers, Cicilia Githaiga, Janeth Calambás, Karen Añaños, Miguel Evanjuanoy Chindoy, Riccardo Vitale, Juan Nelson Rojas, Delores Mondragón, Yuniur Vázquez Rosalío, and Angelina Sacbajá are:

- Reverence
- Respect
- Responsibility
- Relevance
- Regulation
- Reparation
- Restoration
- Reconciliation

Some history: While it might have happened sooner, the dividing line between (a) a few anthropologists finding themselves accepted into tribal gatherings and having these experiences and (b) the actual introduction of a consciousness-altering mushroom to outsiders with no knowledge of the indigenous context, was the year 1955. Shaman María Sabina[59] performed a *velada,* a nighttime healing ceremony with psilocybin mushrooms (probably *Psilocybe mexicana*), and offered those mushrooms to R. Gordon Wasson and those with him.

Wasson promised María Sabina that he would not share the secret of the mushrooms with anyone. Instead, he violated her trust and shared his session (including pictures) with a friend who, in 1957, put the story on the cover of *Life.* This forever changed the lives not only of María Sabina and members of her village but of many others as well.

Wasson also took spores with him. "The fungus was cultivated in Europe and its active ingredient was duplicated as the chemical psilocybin in the laboratory by Albert Hofmann in 1958."[60]

The use of mushrooms for spiritual discovery was not unknown in

Europe; there are a number of medieval churches with remarkable murals of Christ with psychedelic mushrooms.[61] There have been speculative books suggesting that Christianity itself evolved from mushroom experiences not so different from those shared by María Sabina.* Still, it was from the publicity around María Sabina that Westerners became interested in psilocybin-containing mushrooms.

Let's return to the immediate question of cultural appropriation in modern microdosing, which may be easier to understand given this larger history and context.

Modern microdosing did *not* arise from any awareness, understanding, or experience of any indigenous use. It arose from initial suggestions made by Albert Hofmann, the creator of LSD, a substance not found in nature and not previously used in healing, coming-of-age, or divination rituals. LSD is a semisynthetic compound, and it was only thanks to Hofmann's original mistaken overdosing that the assumption came about that the only interesting aspects of LSD were doses twenty to fifty times greater than what we now know to be the range for successful microdosing.

Microdosing began, therefore, without any knowledge of how it might be beneficial. Early guesses, fumbles, mistakes, and reports led to a gradual focusing in on these low doses. Similarly, dose ranges, protocols, and the unique practice of taking weeks off came into place early on.

At one point, Jim convinced himself that he was the one who had discovered the uses of very low doses, forgetting entirely that the idea had come from the little he'd heard of Albert Hofmann's use. Jim was brought down to earth by an anthropologist friend who said, "Don't you think it likely that indigenous groups, using the psychedelic substances available to them, would have tried low doses?" The obviousness of this question ended Jim's fantasy, but did not lead

---

*See, for example, Brian Muraresku's *The Immortality Key* (2020).

him or others to investigate ways in which low doses had already been used. Jim had so little experience at that time that it also hadn't yet occurred to him that a dose correct for one person might not be correct for another.

Sandoz-synthesized psilocybin was the original chemical used by the Harvard Group in the early 1960s for research and extensive personal experimentation until someone showed up from New York City with a jar of LSD. LSD disrupted the entire Harvard community. (After Tim Leary took it for the first time, having previously had many, many experiences with psilocybin, he didn't speak for several days. Ram Dass [then still Richard Alpert] said, "I thought we'd lost Timmy.") The great flowering of psychedelic consciousness across the country was primarily fueled by LSD, not psilocybin or psilocybin-containing mushrooms.*

The first several years of exploration and expanding interest in microdosing focused on LSD. Put differently, it is historically correct to say that microdosing initially began and developed using LSD. As psilocybin mushrooms became more available, most people simply tried to equate dose levels and treat psilocybin exactly as LSD had been treated, without recourse, understanding, or awareness of indigenous use.

Now we are in a different era. While the wider use of psychedelics today encompasses a range of substances, many already used by indigenous cultures for centuries, almost no high-dose research or therapy has tried to integrate their understandings, let alone their tested techniques.

We would like to avoid getting caught up in the argument that because indigenous use preceded current use, current use must in some sense be necessarily exploitive. It may be more beneficial and accurate for all parties to simply hold contemporary microdosing—developed

*The widespread availability of LSD occurred in part because a few clandestine chemists made enough LSD to keep it inexpensive and accessible. Nick Sanders (who served jail time for his production of LSD) recalls that he probably created 250 million doses. There were other chemists as well.

outside indigenous insights or practices—as another set of indigenous practices, that is, indigenous to the individuals and groups who first developed them, the contemporary worldwide microdosing community.

Thus, modern microdosing can be understood as a natural development arising from personal experiences, explored sufficiently to be of use to others. The fundamental experience and effects of microdosing are neither Western nor indigenous, tribal nor religious, but a gift from plants, fungi, and some laboratory-created molecules as well.*

While there is growing worldwide interest in rediscovering ways of using consciousness-altering substances, this book primarily consists of descriptions of current usage, predominantly in Western-dominated cultures, and does not often look to indigenous practices, which differ from group to group and from substance to substance. This is neither a weakness nor a strength; we are simply reporting what has occurred.

We are already starting to see—and in the near future, can expect more of—the blending of Western curiosity and indigenous practice. For example, the Microhausca group based in Peru is comprised of young, educated, scientifically trained and psychologically sophisticated individuals working closely with Shipibo-Conibo[†] shamans. They are developing new methods of using tiny amounts of native plants to alleviate human suffering and open up individuals to a greater awareness of their interdependence with all living things.

That's where we find ourselves. We continue to work together the way nature does, making use of our individual strengths to support one another's contributions. There is no way to undo the horrific damage done to all the peoples of the Americas and other exploited places, but with continued intention and goodwill, we can learn from each other to prevent more damage when possible. As part of that, modern microdosing

---

*We are grateful to María Sabina, who shared ancestral knowledge, and whose life was deeply harmed by so doing. We are also grateful to Albert Hofmann, who first synthesized LSD (and psilocybin).

†The Shipibo-Conibo are an indigenous people who live along the Ucayali River in the Amazon rainforest in Peru.

has joined the worldwide community as another member, adding what it has developed to the extensive already existing knowledge base.

> We are here to make a better world.
> —Abbie Hoffman

First Use of the Term "Microdosing"

Who first used the term "microdosing"?

As just discussed, in some ways the practice of microdosing can be said to go back thousands of years. But as pointed out by the German psychiatrist Torsten Passie in his 2019 book, the term "microdosing" itself was first used as part of "Clearlight Brand 'microdose' LSD," made by Davivid Rose* around forty years earlier. According to Passie:

> If the story about "Clearlight Brand 'microdose' LSD" is true, the origin of the use of the term 'microdose' for very low doses of LSD . . . precedes all other uses of the term, e.g., in pharmacology (since 1995), in agriculture (since 2005) and by Fadiman (2011).[62]

Davivid Rose has extensively documented his own history on Blogspot, Twitter, and Flickr. In his own words:

> The first batch of microdoses I produced were made in Berkeley around 1980 from LSD I illegally purchased. It was called "CLEARLIGHT Brand MIND VITAMIN TABLETS" and came in labeled shrink-wrapped brown glass bottles, each containing 100 tablets. Each tablet contained 100 milligrams of

---

*Neither Jim nor Jordan knew of Davivid Rose's work before this.

ascorbic acid [vitamin C] and 5 micrograms of d-lysergic acid diethylamide. These tablets were given away, not sold.[63]

Davivid Rose's foray into microdosing was a conservative one. The five-microgram dose was less than the seven to twelve micrograms now recommended as the beginning dose range for microdosing LSD. He felt you should not take the microdoses unless you were in the presence of a "willing and experienced guide," and offered the following advice:

> My LSD microdosing instructions: First and most impor-
> tantly, CUT THE CRAP. Then, and only then, should a
> person ever take LSD. (LSD is a nonspecific amplifier. If you
> are full of shit you don't need to amplify your shittiness. If you
> are delusional, you don't need to amplify your delusions.)[64]

Davivid Rose reports that the people who received "the most benefit from the tablets were a major symphony orchestra chorus. MANY of the singers took the tablets over the course of perhaps 6 months, and said their experiences were 'wonderful.'"[65] Such positive experiences were no doubt partly attributable to the instructions that came with "Clearlight Brand 'microdose' LSD"—which was sometimes packaged as part of a coloring book for adults. Rose describes set and setting, recommends a book list, and strongly suggests that people pay great attention to setting up the experience and then take the necessary time—a number of days—to fully integrate it. In many ways, Rose's first go at microdosing embodied much of what we still agree is safe, sensible, and effective. He also had a good idea of the wide range of potential results:

> These squares are amazingly versatile psychic tools that have
> a wide variety of uses. For example, there are numerous ways
> in which these squares may be employed by a bona-fide healer
> to catalyze a balanced physical/mental restructuring. Some
> people consider these squares to be an excellent sacrament if

used in an appropriate religious setting. These squares may also prove to be of great value to an intelligent user who is seriously interested in exploring her or his creative potential.[66]

Following this "proof of concept," Rose obtained enough LSD to make four hundred thousand doses, which he intended, as before, to give away. Unfortunately, law enforcement became aware of his project and seized the entire batch. He was arrested and charged with possession, but avoided any jail time. His attempt to introduce the use of tiny amounts of LSD was over, and while he had indeed called his small doses "microdoses," neither the name nor his generosity have generally been noticed, until now.

Beginning of Modern Microdosing

Why and how did modern microdosing take shape and become widely known?

After Jim's conversation with Bob Forte, described in "Dosage Ranges for Different Substances" in chapter 2—and despite a long career in psychedelics where such low doses had never been of any interest—his curiosity was piqued. He started collecting stories about psychedelic microdosing, and began asking people to send him reports in letters or emails. At one point, after Jim had given a talk at a conference, a stranger came up to him and said:

> "You know what would be really cool? Imagine if someone sent out to people's mailing addresses something like a page, like blotter paper, with little pictures of Hofmann and Janis with ten mics in each picture, along with a pen and a pad so people can take notes. What do you think of that?"

Jim said, "You're asking me if I'm going to be sending drugs illegally through the mail with my return address?" And the fellow said, "No, no, I will!" (The "blotter paper plus instructions" that was sent out included twenty thumbnail images—four rows across and five columns down—each containing ten micrograms, featuring Jim Morrison, Tina Turner, Yoda, John Lennon, Alice from *Alice in Wonderland*, Ram Dass, Jimi Hendrix, Debbie Harry, Rick Doblin, Steve Jobs, Patti Smith, Wavy Gravy, Hunter S. Thompson, Janis Joplin, Jerry Garcia, Barack Obama, Terence McKenna, J. R. "Bob" Dobbs, and of course, Timothy Leary. The bottom half of the page had a simple description of what had been sent out, and then requested a code name, age, gender, and occupation. Stating that "a sentence or two a day is more than enough" for each microdosing session, it noted that any positive or adverse effects on health conditions were of particular interest.) After Jim began receiving quite a few reports, he teamed up with Sophia Korb, who had all the tech, data crunching, and research skills that he lacked.*

Based on his increasing interest and excitement, and the reports he received, Jim's 2011 book, *The Psychedelic Explorer's Guide*, included a chapter called "Can Sub-Perceptual Doses of Psychedelics Improve Normal Functioning?" After that, according to Torsten Passie:

> Interest in microdosing was boosted when Fadiman was interviewed by Tim Ferriss in March 2015. Shortly after the podcast was aired, an article on microdosing appeared in *Rolling Stone* magazine.[67] Journalists picked up on the 'new trend' and began to write articles, which boosted awareness and interest. At first, it was reported that microdosing was limited to some creative workaholics in Silicon Valley, but after a few more articles appeared, its popularity spread significantly.

---

*Early on, Sophia Korb said to Jim, "Why don't we collect this information systematically? We'll just put it out there, and anyone who writes us will get back how to do it safely, how to do it carefully, and also a daily checklist of 'Here's twenty different emotional states; please just check off how you're doing on a regular basis. And at the end of your thirty days, or anytime in between, send us the checklist along with a report of anything that wasn't on the checklist.'" Sophia's innovation and craftsmanship turned Jim's cottage industry efforts into a data collection machine that at one point received forty thousand data points a week.

These other early articles included one by *Forbes* called "LSD Micro-dosing: The New Job Enhancer in Silicon Valley and Beyond,"[68] which came out a week after the *Rolling Stone* article, and one published in *Wired UK* in 2016 called "Under Pressure, Silicon Valley Workers Turn to LSD Microdosing."[69] Microdosing's popularity was then cemented into place with Ayelet Waldman's early 2017 book, *A Really Good Day: How Microdosing Made a Mega Difference in My Mood, My Marriage, and My Life*. Since then, microdosing's popularity has only continued to increase, spread mainly by word of mouth, as well as increasing scientific and public interest generally.

[7]

Conclusions

What's Left Out

This book focuses on what you need to know about microdosing, from basic information and safety concerns to studies and stories embodying best practices of every kind. As a result, in addition to a few areas that we specifically state we wouldn't be covering—like sourcing psychedelics— there are quite a few other areas of relevance and interest that were simply beyond our scope. Here is a partial list of what was left out of this book.

Social Issues: Many economic, cultural, and political considerations— from effects on the environment to social injustice issues—are beyond the scope of this book. Problems and inequities will certainly continue to arise as the psychedelic revival moves forward, but these won't change what we have learned about effective microdosing from participatory citizen science reports and, increasingly, from hard science.

Research Issues: We have reported some of the research on single doses, measured in laboratory settings, showing differences among substances. Sometimes we've also mentioned single high-dose studies because they seemed relevant, but most high-dose research is neither reviewed nor cited.

We've mentioned well-established results in some areas, tentative results in others, and single cases special enough to be focused on. We have not presented research that, while perhaps inherently fascinating, has not translated into useful real-world effects.

Accoutrements and External Support: The appearance of so many commercial offerings of so many types in the last few years goes hand-in-hand with the swift rise of microdosing's popularity. But as stated earlier, we cannot act as a referral service, so we are not recommending—nor for the most part describing, comparing, or evaluating—microdosing apps, workshops, meetups, trainings, coaches, institutions, and so on. These all appeal to ever-changing buyers, users, clients, patients, or members, coming and going while morphing into new shapes and directions. You're on your own here.

Theories: We have stayed away as much as possible from theoretical models that, once taken up, need defending, including animal research models that may or may not extrapolate to human beings. The fact (not often acknowledged) is that they rarely do. While it's enticing to say that the reasons for lifting depression, alleviating pain, improving grades, and having better sex are such and such, we wanted to give you something more like a botanical picture book or illustrated tour guide that gives context to the experience of individuals whose daily lives have been changed by microdosing.

Unknowns: The observational citizen science component of microdosing is necessarily limited to those who felt it was important to share their experiences, often in detail. People we've never heard from may have experienced things very differently than those who shared. While this epistemological conundrum may intrigue researchers, most people just want to know: "Did it help at all?" "Did it help enough to matter?" "Would it possibly help me?"

Throughout the years he has been involved in microdosing—from initial descriptions to early reports, surveys, and conferences, and from individual trainings and coaching to grappling with the implications of reports on conventional therapies and medications—Jim and the rest of the microdosing community have shared what's been working. That's all we can do.

Some Additional Considerations

Preference for Real-Life Evidence: We never lose sight of microdosing being about the use of substances with thousands of years of prior use or, in the case of LSD, millions of individual users partaking multiple times over decades. Relying on people's actual reports of actual conditions and actual changes over other kinds of data is simply the most conservative approach.

There's No There There: The early criticism that microdosing was no more than heightened expectancy or the body's natural healing response almost drew us into the argument. Instead of responding, it was more important to simply report that because of microdosing, someone (a) had recovered from a stroke after years of rehabilitation, or (b) had come up from depression after ten medications had failed, or (c) was no longer having daily migraines.

We've (mostly) controlled what might be considered our righteous indignation at imagining that due solely to placebo effects, the person who felt better must have "done it to themselves." On reflection, this possibility is much more exciting than attributing healing to microdosing! Yet, if microdosing only fooled those folks into healing themselves, everything described in this book would remain the same.*

The Plane Truth: An image we like to use is that we are flying this plane while still building it. Many early assumptions proved wrong, sincere advice was misdirected, and dose levels, protocols, time off

---

*Decades ago, Jim served as the director of the Institute of Noetic Sciences. Staff member Brendan O'Regan, the first director of research, did a study of "spontaneous healings"—people whose recovery was unexpected and against all medical likelihood. One unreported finding was that *none* of these remarkable people saw their healing as spontaneous. They had done enormous work with diet and lifestyle changes, laying on of hands, working with healers, using remedies unknown to their doctors, and more. They felt insulted that their hard work was dismissed by the medical profession, and rightly so.

advised, and recommended substance have all been revised more than once.

We have an abiding interest in encouraging people to alleviate suffering and improve their lives. When people's lived experience does not fit the scientific model, we remind ourselves it's just a model. When people's lived experience does not fit a theological model, contemporary observers are quite comfortable in reminding us that it's just a model. There is more overlap in those two examples than most people notice or acknowledge.

Please consider this book's stories and research as open doors. Some lead nowhere, some lead to better lives, some lead to miracles. You can just peek in; you can stand on the threshold; you can walk through the door; and sometimes, once you're through the door, you may find you're more remarkable than you ever expected.

Predictions

Making predictions is a loser's game. That's why predictions are placed safely at the end of a long book, where they provide entertainment, not serious science or helpful information. They are also a podcast and interview staple—especially if the host knows little about the topic—a softball question to fill a program's last few minutes.

In *The Psychedelic Explorer's Guide,* published in 2011, Jim made a few predictions about the future of psychedelics. One or two were close to the mark, but he missed virtually every major development. Having not learned the lesson, here's what we've got for you.

Greed Accelerates Change

Not foreseen was how the psychedelic revival, with its promise of the possibility of vast profits, would accelerate the creation, manufacture, and distribution of psychedelics, as well as therapeutic and service offerings, spawning new substances, distribution schemes, patent grabs, lawsuits, publicly traded companies, and Wild West speculation. Benefiting humanity is still a consideration, but too often has become secondary.

Microdosing, like the diminutive hobbits Bilbo and Frodo in *The Lord of the Rings*, has been able to diversify and develop by not bringing attention to itself; by not worrying about legislation, patent protections, or medical acceptance; and even by not having much concern about current conventional scientific methodologies (some of which are inappropriate for measuring improvements in subjective states).

The first era of modern microdosing was already ending when we started this book. The high-minded, idealistic, benefits-first people who created the worldwide microdosing community were already being scouted by profiteers looking for ways microdosing could be made more profitable. One avenue being considered is restricting its use to those with special training and licenses.* Similarly, synthesized microdoses could potentially be profitably patented like pharmaceuticals. Early inspired amateurs and citizen scientists are now being supplanted by this next generation of those with certifications, trainings, degrees, and legal permissions. It doesn't take much expertise to predict that things will generally work out better for this new class of owners and experts than for ordinary users.

Will medicalization and professionalization come with social and cultural injustice and exploitation? Will it discriminate against those with fewer opportunities to gain such certifications and legal permissions? Will it come with at least one eye focused on personal gain and attempts to gain market share, whether or not honestly?

Of course it will.

Still, will many people—with or without permission—continue

---

*Just as having a theory forces one into spending time protecting it, expanding its scope, defending it from other theories, and pre-planning research to support it, expertise in the ins and outs of microdosing is quickly becoming competitive. This substance, teacher, institution, retreat, or group is supposedly better for you than that substance, teacher, institution, retreat, or group, and so forth. We have done our best to stick with reporting observations and researching findings while not privileging specific theories or service offerings.

to make cultivated microdoses available, freely giving information to anyone who asks, while exploring and expanding areas where microdosing might be beneficial?

Of course they will.

Substances New and Old

Almost none of the companies eager to profit from psychedelics have noticed microdosing yet. Eventually, they will recognize that having customers take a substance once in a lifetime or a few times a year is not as good a business model as selling something they'll take every few days for weeks or months. Expect entrepreneurial greed, but in slow motion, with the ease of growing mushrooms as a counterforce.

The low cost and variety of mushroom growing kits keeps lowering the price. Underground growers two years ago were getting $1,500 a pound for dried mushrooms; a year ago, it was $1,000. Currently, it is just $250 (at least in Northern California). With the ongoing shift away from the use of LSD or its derivatives toward easily available mushrooms, unregulated use will continue to expand.

Microdosing Coaching and Services

There is already the rise of a new occupational category—"Microdosing Professional"—appealing to individuals already licensed in other healing professions.

One of the best coaches Jim knows—someone who has succeeded with some very difficult physical and mental conditions—was offering a training based on his work with several hundred clients. To his surprise, even before the training officially opened for sign-ups, he was sought out—primarily by licensed health professionals—interested in microdosing within their specialty. There is already an international microdosing professional organization, and there will be national microdosing organizations that more and more will resemble those in other healing specialties.

Dementia Will Turn Out to Be Positively Impacted

This prediction is a long shot, but we believe that microdosing will turn out to have a positive effect on dementia, slowing or stabilizing the decline. It wasn't included in the A to Z conditions list because we have too few reports, but each of these showed a swift uptick in cognition, memory, and mood for a few hours after a single microdose. As with many other possibilities, it may not happen, but we remain optimistic.

The Future Is Already Here

A few more specific predictions:

- The *rise of psychedelic churches*: successfully sidestepping commercial and legislative swamps, these institutions will become a major force within the psychedelic revival as they make available high doses for rituals and services, and microdoses for health and well-being.
- There will *be full-page ads in magazines* like *The New Yorker* for microdoses and microdosing organizations, just as there are now full-page ads for perfume, liquor, and luxury cruises.
- *Varieties of psychedelic mushrooms will be differentiated,* not only by the strength of their alkaloids but by subtle subjective effect differences, as well as differences in texture and taste. As with wine, and more recently coffee and cannabis, there will be extensive offerings of microdoses with new hybrid varieties of mushrooms entering the market seasonally. For microdoses, we will soon see all the facets of modern media-dominated marketing—brands, packaging, influencers—

focused on mushrooms. (As described earlier, early research shows laboratory-created psilocybin is not as effective.)

It's a bit of a cheat to call these predictions, as they are all already beginning to happen. As of this moment (Easter 2024), probably the largest single church in the Bay Area is the Church of Ambrosia, with over 100,000 members. Instead of selling psychedelic products, it offers them to members, along with a suggested donation amount for each listed item.

As for ads, the February 2024 issue of *The New Yorker* had a full-page color ad, with the top third just "Microdosing Psychedelics." Then it describes how, by joining an organization, one will not only have access to psychedelics but will receive a free sample upon becoming a member.

As for the rollout of dozens of underground mushroom-based products, the rush is on. Elegant packaging and variations in color, flavor, and strength are beginning to proliferate. One current favorite is "elixirs" of fresh herbs and dried mushrooms, available in a variety of herbal combinations.

Nicer People Increase Hope and Possibility

The 1960s were characterized by an enormous outburst of activist optimism focused on increasing human happiness and compassion, ending the subjection and suppression of women, and returning to a healthier and more intimate relationship with the natural world.

We may get a second chance. While we recognize and feel the despair over the reality of the possible destruction of civilization, this book is part of another possibility. In a massive understatement, Paul Stamets noted that people who use psychedelics are nicer—nicer to themselves, each other, and the natural world.

To the extent that nicer people proliferate and begin to flourish in science and medicine—and even in politics—it becomes possible to imagine and work toward creating a world in which better health and what it takes to maintain it are considered basic universal rights.

Worldwide, indigenous users of psychedelics often describe their plants or fungi not as medications or intoxicants but as teachers. We are rediscovering ways to learn what we need most, and ways of restoring balance to ourselves, our species, and our habitats. For millennia, microdosing has been one way to become more aware of our relationship with all living beings. Its global growth may be part of nature's way of restoring global harmony. Together, we're working on it.

Jim's Final Reflections

This book completes a circle that began in 2009 when I added a chapter on microdosing to *The Psychedelic Explorer's Guide* (2011).

Written later than the rest of the book, it was a brief introduction to microdosing with a few early reports on the effects being different from higher doses. Only after microdosing had begun to be a topic of interest did the media refer to the chapter as the first published article about microdosing and as seminal in expanding general awareness of microdosing. This book completes that chapter's intentions.

My goal then (as now) was not to share my opinions about how wonderful, complicated, difficult, or special taking microdoses would be for you, or for your mother, or for your best friend. It was to present first-person accounts for you to look over and consider so you could come to your own conclusions.

When we began outlining this book, the research community's complaint about microdosing was that there wasn't enough research to be sure that it had any effects at all—maybe it was all expectation and placebo.

While first-person accounts do not directly respond to those questions, they do encourage further explorations. A major goal I've had from the outset was to interest others in finding out more. My hope is that this book will continue to spur that process. As longtime psychedelic researcher Amanda Feilding said, "We're looking for the right dose for the right conditions."

Formal research is one way to evaluate the validity of accumulated individual experiences, but it is not a substitute for them. There are different ways to climb a mountain, yet the view from the top is the same. To argue about this or that route is to lose track of why you're climbing in the first place.

As I reflect on what we've done with this book, the image that comes to mind is an animal park or botanical garden. In these places, you get to see a wide variety of animals, plants, fungi, or fish without any filter. No theory, no methodology—just your own experience.

We opened one chapter with a wonderful quote from Professor David Nutt, whose skepticism about any treatment or substance that promises to help too many conditions was—we all agreed—a good place to start . . . as well as a good place to end.

I wanted to introduce you to a wider world than you could find on your own, to increase your curiosity, and often, to surprise you. To the extent what you've read has made you wonder about all this, and gets you to keep wondering, this book will have done its job. It has taken you to many different trailheads and describes what we know about each.

Thank you for joining in these discoveries. You now know enough, if you choose, to find a trail and make it your own.

Jordan's Final Reflections

In order for any sort of genuine transformation to occur [there must be] not a new theory or worldview, but a new type of social practice, mode of production, concrete behavioral injunctions, or experimental exemplars.

—Ken Wilber[1]

A scientific truth does not triumph by convincing
its opponents and making them see the light,
but rather because its opponents eventually die
and a new generation grows up that is familiar with it.
—Max Planck

Surprises and Changes

While I've played a substantial role in completing about three dozen books in forty years of professional writing and editing, this project was like none other.

From the importance and promise of the subject matter, to the intensity of integrating waves of new information in real time—especially as manuscript deadlines approached—an ever-evolving mélange of new studies, self-reports, and real-world developments had to be dealt with.

Giving myself fully to this process changed me in ways I can see, and no doubt, in ways I can't. It taught me things that surprised me, and clarified three personal core takeaways that end this reflection.

It also renewed my faith in the ability of all of us to help each other as we collectively open ourselves to the support of these natural medicines and their derivatives and analogues. Having so many people contribute to our efforts, share information, give leads or reports on unusual conditions, help us reframe our thinking, and just cheer us on was extraordinarily gratifying. Simultaneously, as we continued to write, we shared our new knowledge—both what we knew and what we didn't—with friends and acquaintances, so others could make better decisions for themselves.

In the end, it all came together. We worked out what needed to be said about difficult or controversial areas, and found ways to gently but firmly address early claims that with microdosing "there's no real effect." Finally, it became clear that the manuscript was truly synergistic—that is, the intensive effort needed to comprehensively bring together what's known about modern microdosing resulted in a work that was and is greater than the sum of its parts.

Human Potential and the Potential of Microdosing

With psychedelics, while the big news, big money, and big focus remain on higher doses, in some ways, microdosing may be potentially more revolutionary—more of a "disruptor" of the status quo*—one that obviously, desperately, needs upgrading.

When I interned for a Ralph Nader–inspired public interest group (NYPIRG) during college, the realization came to me that "politics as usual was doomed," and the only possible way to change things—the only way to save our planet, Gaia, which by then, thanks to psychedelics, I had a personal relationship with—was to find ways to reliably access and better deploy human potential.[†]

About thirty years after that college epiphany, I first heard about microdosing from Jim. At that point in my life, I was focused on making good things better, that is, on enhancing my wellness, abilities, and flow. No one, including me, imagined then that microdosing could affect particular health conditions, and certainly not the A to Z list we've described here.

How things have changed! Microdosing has a demonstrated ability to unlock and unleash human potential in a wide range of areas, from healing to improved functioning. To help unlock and unleash your own potential using microdosing, here are my three core takeaways.

---

*Compared to using macrodoses, microdosing is far less expensive, far less complicated, far safer, and remarkably robust in the positive outcomes being produced, for mental and physical health conditions and for enhanced abilities, wellness, and flow.

†Inspired by Aldous Huxley, Timothy Leary, Robert Anton Wilson, Charles Tart, Jean Houston, John Curtis Gowan, Bill Eichman, and many others, I continued my personal search for the extraordinary. As one aspect of this, psychedelics were part of my life, not in an extravagant way but generally at the right times, in the right places, and with the right people.

Takeaway 1: Start by Following the Rules

Microdosing has a set of basic rules, suggestions, or injunctions about dosage level, protocols ("schedules"), and time off. As Ken Wilber put it in the quote opening this reflection, there really is a need for "a new type of social practice . . . concrete behavioral injunctions, or experimental exemplars"—just what we've described in the practical parts of this book.

In the *Saturday Night Live* treatment of microdosing on February 3, 2024, Ayo Edebiri and Mikey Day are a pair of ultra-wholesome college students who become very upset when they find out that their friend Zachary (Andrew Dismukes) is "high" on microdosing after eating a mushroom chocolate. About forty seconds in, Zachary says, "Never done it before, and the hype is real." That's exactly right—the hype is real—especially if at first you follow the rules consciously, closely, and conservatively. As we say throughout, with microdosing, "less is more." (Yes, there are exceptions, but they are rare.)

Even though there is much we still don't know, compared to fifteen years or so ago, when modern microdosing was just getting started, we've learned a great deal. To not take advantage of our collective knowledge base, and the rules and practices that generally work for most people, is simply to shoot yourself in the foot. No need to make mistakes that can be easily avoided.

Takeaway 2: The Science Is Already Here

The science Q&As were among the last parts of the book we finished. Figuring out what needed to be said and how to say it was challenging, both because of incomplete and evolving information and because we were proposing an alternative take on certain types of science. Specifically, substantial observational science shows, without doubt, that the phenomenon is real—in the sense of making a difference for people and improving their lives.

Areas of current scientific controversy are addressed in their own write-ups in chapter 6. Of course, there are good reasons to be, and remain, skeptical. But there are better reasons to be flexible and open-minded when thousands upon thousands of community-based citizen science observations show so clearly how many people have already had powerful and sustained results.

Major concerns—including the potential for triggering psychosis or causing heart valve damage—have vanishingly little if any actual factual basis or support behind them. Additionally, we now know for certain, across a variety of tests, that microdosing produces the same general physiological signatures as macrodosing, just at a lower amplitude.

When the double-blind randomized placebo criteria are inappropriately applied, they often fail to capture the effects of microdosing. As Jeff Bezos concisely states at the start of chapter 6, this usually means that standard science is simply measuring the wrong thing. At the very least, it's fair to say that when studying microdosing, observational science is often more germane than double-blind placebo-controlled randomized studies (originally instituted by legislation created to improve the safety of new pharmaceuticals). Claims that microdosing results are based solely on expectations have, as well, fallen by the wayside as new research comes to light.

Takeaway 3: The Signal We're Collectively Generating Is Growing Ever Stronger

When Jim started focusing on microdosing around 2010, even though the signal he first collected and put together was relatively weak, the overall efficacy and value of the practice quickly became apparent. As he pulled in more stories, ideas, and then scientific studies, the signal was amplified, making it clearer and easier for others to find—a positive feedback loop or (in this case, a truly) virtuous cycle.

That signal became even stronger once Jim wrote the chapter on microdosing in *The Psychedelic Explorer's Guide* (2011), and was then additionally strengthened through conference appearances, magazine articles, and interviews, thereby attracting more self-reports and studies, further amplifying the signal, and so on. All this ultimately led to this book. Now, with an A to Z health conditions list of around thirty-five topics, and a wide variety of ways of enhancing abilities, wellness, and flow coming into focus, the signal is stronger than ever.

When modern microdosing is fifty years old, in 2060, will it still be recognizable as defined in this book? Based on the strength of the signal presented here, I'm guessing "yes," with a few provisos:

- Our knowledge base will have substantially and perhaps dramatically expanded.
- Some things we thought we knew will turn out to have been wrong.
- A large number of additional health conditions addressed—as well as ways of enhancing abilities, wellness, and flow—will have emerged and been documented, coupled with the rise of associated interest groups and organizations (nonprofit and for profit).

If we do arrive at a point where microdosing becomes widely practiced and correctly appreciated, this will have only been made possible through our combined efforts and ingenuity, and because of our collective willingness to take chances, experience things for ourselves, and give back to the community what we've learned. As individuals, the small steps we take may seem insignificant, but they are not. By taking small steps together—hand-in-hand, heart-in-heart, vision upon vision—we can build unstoppable collective momentum on the path to a better world.

Acknowledgments

Jim

This book was only possible through the generosity of thousands of people who submitted reports about their own experiences—especially the many quoted here—all of whom were promised that they would not be given individual credit for their contributions. Promise kept.

Thanks to those groups and individuals (not directly linked to microdosing) who created and extended the psychedelic revival, which—indirectly and usually inadvertently—also supported the development of microdosing. Thanks also to the worldwide underground of guides and growers whose determination to alleviate suffering couldn't wait until science is convinced and governments allow full use.

Thanks to:

My wonderful friend Jordan, who was responsible for so much more than the writing, keeping us both on track, never letting a sentence go by without ensuring it was as clear and as accurate as possible, and who, ever so gently, pulled me back to center whenever I'd lose my cool completely.

Our better-than-we-could-have-imagined editor, Elizabeth Beier, who improved every aspect of our writing; her ultra-reliable assistant,

Brigitte Dale, who helped us through many at first seemingly impossible technical challenges; and our agent, James Levine, who made it possible to work with this team in the first place.

My wife, Dorothy, who supported not only this work but me personally in every way possible during the several years it took to put this book together, and for the many decades she has continued to make it possible for me to do what I needed to do throughout many earlier jobs, books, and projects; and my two daughters, Renee and Maria, both gifted teachers and endlessly supportive.

My small dogs, Timmie and Adam, who, over the last twelve years, have reminded me that I am not special and still can be loved. I remain amazed how often their daily grounding keeps reopening my heart and saving me from losing my way.

The small group of healers whose expertise I leaned on when I regularly exceeded my own capacity to do this work: Rachael Henrichsen, Richard Baldwin, Scott Wood, David St. Claire, Connie Hernandez, Seth Weisman, Jamie Paychev, and Dave Rabin.

Thanks to the numerous clinicians, researchers, scientists, and journal editors who considered, observed, speculated, tested, analyzed, reported on, or scoffed at microdoses and microdosing. Your contributions served to validate and support the necessity for the explorations of individual experiences that are the core of this book.

Thanks especially to those researchers who opened up, verified, or clarified novel or unique aspects of psychedelic research in general, and microdosing in particular. First and foremost, my partner early on, Sophia Korb Cohon, who helped me move past stacking up piles of reports in boxes to conducting the first online worldwide (fifty-one countries) microdosing exploration.

Thanks to so many others: Amanda Feilding, Nick Cozzi, Conor Murray, Harriet de Wit, Roland Griffiths, Suresh Muthukumaraswamy, Vince Polito, Mariana Zarankin, Julie Holland, Gathering Wind, Mark Haden, Albert Garcia-Romeu, Charles Grob, Aaron Orsini, Andrew Kornfeld, David Nutt, Baba Masha, Boris Heffets, James

Keim, Natasha Mason, Rotem Petranker, Thomas Anderson, and Emmanuelle Schindler. Extra gratitude to the team at Quantified Science who let me be part of their launching the largest and most diverse set of microdose surveys to date, including Joseph Rootman, Pamela Kryskow, Kalin Harvey, Eesmyal Santos-Brault, Kim P. C. Kuypers, Francoise Bourzat, and Zach Walsh, and especially Paul Stamets, known for numerous scientific breakthroughs related to psilocybin mushrooms and microdosing. Along with Jim Warren, Paul encouraged and supported my research when I most needed affirmation.

Thanks to:

Those scientists, researchers, and even some commercial companies that raised critical questions leading us to evaluate the most basic premises about microdose effects. Thank you, Torsten Passie, Robin Carhart-Harris, David Nichols, Charles Nichols, Kelan Thomas, and Balázs Szigeti.

Hein Pijnnaken, Jakobien van der Weijden, Brittany Lillegard, and all the staff and volunteers at the Microdosing Institute in Holland who helped develop much of the initial framework referred to throughout this book for safe successful preparations and ways of use.

Álvaro Zárate and Adolfo Schmitt, who founded Microhuasca in Peru (focusing on microdosing protocols and programs with ayahuasca and other sacred medicines), and who have helped create and support several dozen independent microdosing groups throughout Latin America.

Tim Ferriss, Sam Harris, and many print journalists and podcast hosts who helped me say more clearly what I was doing and why. Lucy Walker, the footage you used in Michael Pollan's Netflix special included the quote on the book's cover, for which no amount of thanks can be enough. Also, filmmakers Maria Fernandes and Nicole Pritchett for their work in progress, as well as Shelby Hartman at *DoubleBlind*, Jamie Ducharme at *Time*, and C. J. Spotswood, whose book helped health professionals understand microdosing's potential.

Kathy Ushiba for all things tech, recovering lost drafts, and way more.

Bob Wold and his organization, Clusterbusters, who pioneered participatory citizen science by successfully developing treatments for cluster headaches.

A deep bow of gratitude to Adam Bramlage, who—while becoming one of the first microdose coaches and now a teacher of coaches—has been there for me in endless ways. By working with conditions that I doubted microdosing could help, to my delight, Adam keeps proving me wrong.

I've been blessed by companions along the way who did so much work during the long pause between the early work in the sixties and the current revival: Bob Jesse, Rick Doblin, Andy Weil, Ralph Metzner, Stan Grof, Peter Webster, and Michael Murphy; as well as numerous chemists who risked prison to allow a whole generation to come to their own conclusions; the many members of the free-floating community that traveled with the Grateful Dead; and the tens of thousands who create an alternate reality every year at Burning Man. Bouquets of flowers for Diane Darling, who revivified the Guild of Guides, a still-invisible organization, giving many who had worked in isolation a forum to meet, teach, and support one another.

Special friends whose contributions defy categorization include Jill Mellick, Madelyn Cooper, Rachel and Andrew, James Evans, Mary Apra, Jerry Stolaroff, Tim Doody, Shane LeMaster, Daniel Carcillo, Gwylim Llwydd, Melinda Welker, Jeanette Delmar, and so many others.

A final and heartfelt honoring of Robert Forte, who said of microdosing, "I told many people about it, but Jim Fadiman was the only one who ran with it."

Jordan

Just as a large network of people who contributed their precious stories and experiences made the creation of modern microdosing itself possible, this book would not exist without the network of personal friendships and relationships that brought together so many essential elements. Through my old friend Steve McIntosh I became friends with Carter

Phipps and Ellen Daly, and through Ellen, Jim and I were connected to our exceptional agent, James Levine. He kept his promise to serve as a full-fledged intellectual partner, not just an agent. His insight that a focused but friendly question-and-answer format might be best . . . proved exactly correct.

Our completely revised proposal in Q&A format caught the enthusiastic attention of several top publishers, and our choice to work with executive editor Elizabeth Beier of St. Martin's Publishing Group has proven incredibly fruitful. Elizabeth, from her very first read, poured her full attention and bountiful mind into what we'd written—questioning, prodding, suggesting, revising, and injecting a powerful spirit of balanced inquiry into our process. Associate editor Brigitte Dale also proved immensely helpful, especially on otherwise overwhelming technical challenges. We are also grateful to St. Martin's Publishing Group for the copyediting, publicity, marketing, and technical publishing assistance provided by Amelia Beckerman, Brant Janeway, Angus Johnston, John Karle, Melanie Sanders, Jennifer Rohrbach, and Anne Marie Tallberg. We're a great team, and it's a pleasure to work together.

As for overcoming technical challenges, our friends network also brought us James McConchie, who provided our wonderful cover art images (and who has made a difference to this book and my life in many ways); Rebecca Glazer (whose mother, Robin Kohn, has often offered me a thoughtful, kind ear), who brought reliability, form, and precision to our references and footnotes; and Sandra Dreisbach, who generously helped us forge a more thoughtful and thorough set of disclaimers. We were also fortunate to collaborate with Mikaela de la Myco and Naomi Tolson, who generously allowed us to publish some of their detailed survey research on women's health.

No writer is an island. I would like to effusively and humbly thank my family and close friends for their support. It took everything I had to finish this book, and it just wouldn't have happened without the many people (and several pets) who kept pouring their love, energy, and attention into me.

I owe so much to my family: to my wife, Gail, for her unwavering support and insightful feedback, and being by my side for more than thirty-five years of wonderful marriage; to our daughter, Diana, for her no-holds-barred input on content and style; to Mitch, for his good listening skills, book industry experience, and keen mind; and especially to Linda, who kept me physically and emotionally nourished every single day, and who provided me with continuous content feedback and emotional regulation, especially when the going got tough. And of course, gratitude to our cats and chickens, including those who passed during the book-writing process (we miss you, Fluffy Noir). Together, all of you helped me stay grounded and for the most part relatively well balanced and sane throughout, including during the difficult period when my beloved and sorely missed mother, Lola Gruber, left this earth in 2022. (Mom, if you're aware of this book, I hope it makes you proud.)

Deserving special mention is Billy (Sunshine) Gorson, who was on the phone with me nearly every day providing deep listening, unwavering support, and strategic cajoling. I'd also like to acknowledge the ongoing support of the SpiritMen—Andy, Dave, Ken, Luther, and Tom—whose gentle but astute inquiry and unwavering support always make a big difference. Thanks also to Max Taylor, whose research skills were once again crucial; Liz Elms, who helped keep my body together; Jackson Stock, for your inspiration; and to Jeff Lane, Neil Nitzberg, Marty Lupowitz, Marissa (and the memory of Bill) Eichman, Amy Hallman, David Chilcott, Joy Daniels, Erik Davis, Gabriel DeWitt, Brooklyn Cook and Anish Dutta, Helene and Barry Gruber, Jeramy and Molly Hale, Amber Seitz, and Rachel Marjanovich, just for being there and being part of my life.

Let's have even more bouquets of flowers for our departed wise friend and numinous muse, Diane Darling. Thanks also to Dave Rabin, Paul Austin, and Jim Jenkins and the Discovery Sessions staff for providing Jim and me with public venues for discussing our ideas.

As for my Clubhouse and other psychedelically and spiritually oriented friends, including those of you directly cited throughout as content experts, taken together you made it possible for this book's content to be as cutting-edge and up-to-date as possible, and one way or another, you all made a difference. Thank you to Lauren Alderfer, Ēlen Awalom, Baabaa Baa, Leah Benjamin, Hillary Blair, Bruno Bowmore, John Cannon, Melissa Cauley, Laura Dawn, Carla Detchon, Sandra Dreisbach, Avi Ester, Paulmarq Francois, Norman Fried, Bailey Gimbel, Manesh Girn, Dana Harvey, Marc Hayford, Liz Hoff, Melinda Hogvard, Marc Homer, Patrick Ironwood, Bobby Israel, Robin Jaffe (who made it all possible), Sally Adnams Jones, Dena Justice, Brian and Hephzibah Kaplan, Gregory Landsman, Daniel and Ana Levin, Phoenix MacGregor, Natasha Mantler, Cesar Marin, Harrison and Taylor Meagher, Al Meen, Severiano Mendoza (whose real-world friendship I so greatly value), Danielle Nova, NeuronsToNirvana, Scottie Oceano, Eric Reynolds, Alyssa Riccio, Jen Peer Rich, Daniel Rieders, Macha Shewolf, Wendy Perkins Shoef, Adam Shumays, Martin Stewart, Heron Stone, Danny and Vanessa Panzella-Velez, Catherine Wilke, Michael Wilson, Cole and Tah Witty, and Adam Wright. So many of you have become true (and in some cases, real-world) friends, which means so much to me.

Finally, I'd like to deeply thank Jim, not just for trusting me with the valuable material in this and our previous book but for being open to the profound friendship that has developed between us and sustained us throughout.

Appendix

Medications and Supplements So Far Reported As Safe When Microdosing

James Fadiman, PhD, and Sophia Korb, PhD, originally compiled a list of medications, supplements, and drugs found *not* to cause any adverse or undesirable effects when combined with microdosing. Initially found at MicrodosingPsychedelics.com/what-is-microdosing, the list and any updates are now in the hands of the Microdosing Institute of the Netherlands. What you see here was what was on their website as we went to publication.

Note of Caution

This list does not guarantee that microdosing is safe or effective in combination with the listed medications.

Specifically:

- This list applies to microdosing with LSD and psilocybin only. Other microdosing substances may or may not combine well with your medication or supplements.

- If you take two or more medications, or have a somatic illness or a mental health condition, it is advised to consult a psychiatrist or other medical doctor who is well versed in psychedelics and medication interactions prior to microdosing.

Always consult your MD or psychiatrist if you want to combine, taper off, or discontinue any of your medications.

What if my medication is not on the list?

If your medication is not on this list, it means there is insufficient data to support that microdosing is safe and effective. In this case, please consult a psychiatrist or other medical doctor knowledgeable about psychedelics and medication interactions prior to microdosing.

Painkillers
- Acetaminophen/paracetamol (Tylenol)
- Aspirin
- Codeine
- Dihydrocodeine (Co-dydramol)
- Hydrocodone (Vicodin, Norco)
- Ibuprofen (Advil, Motrin)
- Naproxen (Aleve)
- ~~Tramadol (Ultram)~~
  Do not microdose while taking Tramadol

Heart/high blood pressure medication
- Amiodarone (Cordarone, Nexterone)
- Hydrochlorothiazide (HCTZ, HCT)
- Lisinopril (Prinivil, Zestril)
- Losartan (Cozaar)
- Spironolactone (Aldactone)
- Telmisartan (Micardis, Actavis)
- Valsartan (Diovan)
- Ramipril (Tritace)

Birth control
- Aubra
- Hormonal pills
- Marvelon
- Mirena
- NuvaRing
- Tricyclen

Antacid
- Ranitidine (Zantac)

Antibiotics
- Clindamycin (Cleocin, Dalacin, Clinacin)
- Doxycycline
- Minocycline (Minocin, Minomycin, Akamine)
- Penicillin (Bicillin)

Antifungal
- Fluconazole (Diflucan, Celozole)

Focus medication (ADHD/ADD)
- Amphetamine (Adderall)
- Bupropion (Wellbutrin)
- Dextroamphetamine (Dexedrine, Metamina, Attentin, Zenzedi, Procentra, Amfexa)
- Lisdexamfetamine (Vyvanse)
- Methylphenidate (Ritalin, Biphentin)
- Modafinil (Provigil)

Sleeping
- Zopiclone (Zimovane, Imovane)

- Melatonin
- Zolpidem (Ambien, Stilnox)

Antihistamines
- Cetirizine (Zyrtec)
- Diphenhydramine (Benadryl, Gravol)
- Loratadine (Claritin)
- Ranitidine (Zantac)

Benzodiazepines (anxiety, sleep, seizure)
- Alprazolam (Xanax)
- Clonazepam (Klonopin)
- Diazepam (Valium)
- Flurazepam (Staurodorm)
- Lorazepam (Ativan)

Other anxiolytics
- Etizolam
- Propranolol

Parkinson's medications
- Levodopa
- Pramipexole

Cholesterol medications
- Atorvastatin (Lipitor)
- Rosuvastatin (Crestor)
- Simvastatin (Zocor)
- Statins

Racetams
- Aniracetam
- Phenylpiracetam
- Piracetam

Mood stabilizers and antipsychotics
- Aripiprazole (Abilify)
- Buspirone (Buspar)
- Lamotrigine (Lamictal)
- ~~Lithium~~
  Do not microdose while taking lithium
- Quetiapine (Seroquel)

Diabetes
- Metformin (Glucophage)

Anticonvulsants
- Baclofen (Lioresal)

- Carbamazepine (Tegretol)
- Cyclobenzaprine (Flexeril)
- Gabapentin
- Mirtazapine
- Sodium valproate
- Tizanidine (Zanaflex)
- Primidone
- Topiramate

Thyroid medication
- Methimazole or Thiamazole

Antidepressants
- Bupropion (Wellbutrin)
- Citalopram (Celexa)
- Desvenlafaxine (Pristiq)
- Doxepin (Sinequan)
- Duloxetine (Cymbalta)
- Escitalopram (Lexapro)
- Paroxetine (Paxil)
- Ranitidine (Zantac)
- Sertraline (Zoloft)
- Venlafaxine (Effexor)

Breathing (asthma, COPD)
- Salbutamol (Albuterol)
- Cetirizine (Zyrtec)
- Beclometasone (Clenil Modulite)
- Montelukast (Singulair)

Antiviral
- Nitazoxanide

Recreational drugs
- Alcohol
- Amphetamine (speed)
- Heroin
- Kratom
- Marijuana (cannabis)
- Nicotine

Anti-inflammatory
- Mesalazine (Octasa)

Immunosuppressant
- Hydroxychloroquine (Quensyl)

Erectile Dysfunction
- Tadalafil (Cialis)

Alcohol dependence treatments
- Acamprosate (Campral)
- Disulfiram (Antabuse)
- Naltrexone

Hormones and Steroids
- Norethindrone acetate
- Ethinyl estradiol
- Prednisone (Deltasone, Liquid Pred, Orasone, Adasone, Deltacortisone)
- Estrogen (Premarin)
- Progesterone (Prometrium, Utrogestan, Endometrin)
- Testosterone
- Levothyroxine (Synthroid)
- Naturethroid

GERD
- Esomeprazole (Nexium)
- Pantoprazole (Protonix)
- Dexamethasone

DHEA
- Spironolactone (Aldactone)

Supplements
- 5-HTP
- Albizia
- Ashwagandha
- B100
- BCAAs
- Biotin
- Brahmi
- Bromelain
- Caffeine
- Calcium
- Cayenne
- Chaga
- Chlorophyll
- Choline
- CILTEP
- CoQ10
- Cordyceps
- Creatine
- Eleuthero

- EPA/DHA
- Fish oil
- Ginseng
- Glucosamine
- Iodine
- Iron
- Kelp
- Kratom
- L-theanine
- Lemon balm
- Lion's mane
- Maca
- Magnesium
- MCT
- Methyl sulfonyl methane (MSM)
- Milk thistle
- Multivitamins
- Omega 3/6/9
- Passionflower
- Phosphatidyl
- Probiotics
- Pycnogenol
- Reishi
- Rhodiola
- Rosacea
- Selenium
- Shatavari
- Skullcap
- St. John's wort
- Taurine
- Tulsi
- Turmeric (curcumin)
- Turkey's tail
- Twynsta
- Vitamins
  - B6
  - B12
  - D3
  - K
  - C
  - K2
  - D
- Zinc
- Zinium

Notes

1: Overview

1. The first influential written piece on modern microdosing was a chapter in Jim's 2011 book, *The Psychedelic Explorer's Guide: Safe, Therapeutic and Sacred Journeys* (Inner Traditions).
2. "Microdosing," Wikipedia.
3. "Investigation of Illnesses," U.S. Food and Drug Administration.
4. "Benefits of Microdosing," Microdosing Institute.
5. Ona and Bouso, "Placebo Effect," 194–203.

2: Basics

1. One Jim found useful is D. M. Weisberg's *Cannabis Roadmap: Medical Marijuana Guide for Optimal Health and Wellness* (2023). Jordan recommends *The Cannabis Health Index: Combining the Science of Medical Marijuana with Mindfulness Techniques to Heal 100 Chronic Symptoms and Diseases* (2015) by Uwe Blesching.
2. N. Cozzi, email message to Jim Fadiman, 2020.
3. Hatton et al., "Human Cell Count and Size Distribution."
4. Spotswood, *The Microdosing Guidebook*, 25.
5. See https://en.wikipedia.org/wiki/Legal_status_of_psilocybin_mushrooms for updated information.
6. "Drug Scheduling," United States Drug Enforcement Administration.
7. "Microdosing Psilocybin with Cacao," Pure Kakaw.

8. Rootman et al., "Psilocybin Microdosers."

9. Wietstock, "Lemon Tek."

10. McElory, "Average Magic Mushroom."

11. The description of microdosing with *B. caapi* comes from the internal document "Incremental Calibration and Dosing Method Used by Microhuasca," developed by Microhuasca co-founder Adolfo Schmitt.

12. "Guide to Microdosing *Banisteriopsis caapi*," Microdosing Institute.

13. Wilcox, "Microdosing LSA."

14. Garcia-Romeu et al., "Optimal Dosing for Psilocybin Pharmacotherapy," 353–61.

15. u/Ok_Elevator6365, "Microdosing journey ends with Psychosis."

16. u/Ok_Elevator6365.

17. https://uswebshop.miraculix-lab.com/product/psilo-qtest.

18. Marks et al., "Microdosing Psychedelics Under Local, State, and Federal Law," 573–641.

19. For another well-thought-out look at protocols, see what the Microdosing Institute has to say at https://microdosinginstitute.com/how-to/microdosing-protocols.

20. Ona and Bouso, "Placebo Effect," 194–203.

21. Grabski, "Can Microdosing Psychedelics Improve Your Mental Health?"

22. Cormier, "No Link Found Between Psychedelics and Psychosis."

23. Smith, "Psychedelics Are a Promising Therapy."

24. The most complete and up-to-date version of this list, initially developed by Jim Fadiman and Sophia Korb at MicrodosingPsychedelics.com, is now expanded and managed by the Microdosing Institute of the Netherlands.

25. Bansal et al., "Antidepressant Use."

26. Jaeger, "Psychedelic Mushroom Spores Are Federally Legal."

27. Lieber, "Working Woman's Newest Life Hack."

28. Anonymous, "The Secret to My Successful Career."

29. Bestselling books like Bessel van der Kolk's *The Body Keeps the Score: Brain, Mind, and Body in the Healing of Trauma* (2014) and Gabor Mate's *When the Body Says No: Exploring the Stress-Disease Connection* (2011) have helped lead the way in focusing on working with trauma and stress.

30. Rabin, "Feeling Safe Is the Key to Learning."

31. "Social Connectedness," Centers for Disease Control and Prevention.

32. https://royalsociety.org/about-us/history/#.

33. Jay, *Psychonauts: Drugs and the Making of the Modern Mind.*

3: Enhanced Abilities, Wellness, and Flow

1. Note that positive uses were behind some of microdosing's earliest publicity, as discussed in "Beginning of Modern Microdosing" on page 272.

2. Leonard, "Hot New Business Trip."

3. Fink, "When Silicon Valley Takes LSD."

4. Eubanks, "My Experience Microdosing to Learn a Language." This post has since been removed from Medium.

5. u/KaFaraqGatri07, "What better for language learning?"

6. Anonymous (u/anon3348), "From my personal experience, mushroom microdosing gives you a lot of energy and focus," April 4, 2016, comment on "Microdosing for language learning?" r/Shrooms, Reddit, https://www.reddit.com/r/shrooms/comments/4dc8xp/comment/d1q1fbp. The account that originated this thread has since been deleted.

7. Love, "Long-Lost Best Friends."

8. Haigney, "Psychedelics and Longevity."

9. Haigney.

10. r/Microdosing, Reddit.

11. r/Microdosing.

12. Allen, "LSD Increases Sleep Duration."

13. Latifi, "Social Drug of 2024."

14. R.H. personal correspondence with Jim Fadiman.

15. R.H.

16. u/man_bear_pig_2, "Microdosing for sports performance, my experience."

17. Andersson and Kjellgren, "Twenty Percent Better."

18. McKenna, "Joe Rogan on Micro-dosing Psilocybin."

4: Current Findings of Special Interest

1. Haijen, Hurks, and Kuypers, "Self-Medicate for ADHD."

2. Hutten et al., "Self-Rated Effectiveness of Microdosing."

3. Haijen, Hurks, and Kuypers, "Trait Mindfulness and Personality Characteristics."

4. Ducharme, "Demand for ADHD Drugs."

5. Sibley et al., "Sudden Increases in U.S. Stimulant Prescribing," 571–74.

6. *Week* Staff, "ADHD: The Trouble with Diagnosis."

7. Klayman, *Take Your Pills.*

8. "What Is ADHD?" Centers for Disease Control and Prevention.

9. Danielson et al., "Trends in Stimulant Prescription Fills."

10. Resmovits, "ADHD Is Now Classified as a Specific Disability."

11. Quoted in "Number of People Taking ADHD Drugs," Citizens Commission on Human Rights International.

12. Watson, Clark, and Tellegen, "PANAS Scales," 1063–70.

13. Zarankin, Pellegrini, and Zenteno, "Psilocybin Fungi Microdose Treatment," 33–39.

14. Zarankin et al.

15. Zarankin et al.
16. Fried, "52 Symptoms of Major Depression," 191–97.
17. Quoted in Sanders, "Chemical Imbalance Doesn't Explain Depression."
18. Sanders.
19. Moncrieff and Horowitz, "Chemical Imbalance."
20. "Low Serotonin Levels," UCL News.
21. Ghaemi, "Serotonin Hypothesis."
22. Moncrieff and Horowitz, "Chemical Imbalance."
23. Quoted in Sanders, "Chemical Imbalance Doesn't Explain Depression."
24. Sanders.
25. Much of our information came from sources and interviews in Laura Sanders's February 2023 *Science News* article, "Chemical Imbalance Doesn't Explain Depression."
26. Sanders.
27. Ducharme, "Long COVID Patients Are Reporting Suicidal Thoughts."
28. Ducharme, "Latest Promising Long COVID Treatment."
29. Ducharme, "Long COVID Recovery Remains Rare."
30. Ducharme, "Long COVID Recovery Remains Rare."
31. Numerous clinical studies show all these conditions occur with long COVID.
32. Bonnelle et al., "Analgesic Potential of Macrodoses and Microdoses," 619–31.
33. Bonnelle.
34. Sherman et al., "Real-World Evidence," 2293–97.
35. Reports gathered by Mikaela de la Myco with support from Naomi Tolson and others, in their extensive Mothers of the Mushroom survey. (Mothers of the Mushroom is a cooperative that focuses on research and resources for psychedelic families. See www.mushwomb.love/mothersofthemushroom.)
36. "Microdosing While Breastfeeding," Microdosing Institute.
37. Microdosing Institute.
38. Microdosing Institute.
39. Spotswood, *The Microdosing Guidebook*, 142.
40. Mikaela de la Myco Zoom interview with Jordan Gruber on February 13, 2024.

5: Health Conditions Positively Affected

1. Nutt, *Psychedelics*, 237.
2. "Eating Disorder Statistics," South Carolina Department of Mental Health.
3. "*Amanita muscaria*," Clinton Courier.
4. Lewis-Healy, "Psychedelics Could Eventually Treat Asthma."
5. Braman, "Global Burden of Asthma."
6. Masha, *Microdosing with Amanita Muscaria*, 50.
7. Ulrich, "10 Possible Side Effects."

8. Neiloufar Family et al., "Safety, Tolerability, Pharmacokinetics, and Pharmaco-dynamics," 841–53.

9. Masha, *Microdosing with Amanita Muscaria,* 50.

10. "The word 'neurotypical' may be used to refer to individuals who think, learn, and behave in ways that are considered the norm" (Rudy, 2023).

11. Jewell, "Difference Between Asperger's and Autism."

12. Fadiman, *The Psychedelic Explorer's Guide,* 80.

13. "Eating Disorders," National Institute of Mental Health.

14. See, e.g., Gupta, "Bipolar 1 vs. 2."

15. "Bipolar Disorder," National Institute of Mental Health.

16. Nierenberg et al., "Diagnosis and Treatment of Bipolar Disorder," 1370–80.

17. "Experience with micro-dosing psilocybin," Reddit; u/Connect_Swim_81280, "Microdosing for bipolar 2/ADHD"; u/lolfuys, "Effects of psilocybin mushrooms on bipolar disorder"; u/SteRoPo, "Psilocybin microdosers demonstrate greater observed improvements in mood."

18. Finney, "Is Smoking Weed Bad for Your Heart?"

19. Petrilli et al., "Cannabis Potency," 736–50.

20. "What Is Cerebral Palsy?" Centers for Disease Control and Prevention.

21. Their website (in July 2023) reads, "Everyone is different, and the effects of psilocybin will be different for everyone. A wise approach is to start with a very small dose, perhaps a quarter or half a gram, and adjust it upwards as necessary" (Busting Protocol, 2023).

22. Some of this information was gleaned from a talk on the Clubhouse audio app in a room sponsored by Dana Harvey's Flourish Academy (https://flourishacademy .ca/), with Clusterbusters' executive director Bob Wold and president Eileen Brewer present.

23. "Treatment of Cluster Headache," Clusterbusters.

24. Vandergriendt, "Persistent Postural-Perceptual Dizziness."

25. "What Is Persistent Postural Perceptual Dizziness?" Ménière's Society.

26. "What Is Eczema?" National Eczema Association.

27. "Psilocybin and Epilepsy," Sanctuary Wellness Institute.

28. Masha, *Microdosing with Amanita Muscaria,* 58.

29. There have been increasing numbers of clinical studies and trials investigating the use of CBD (cannabidiol) for treating certain types of epilepsy. These include: Devinsky, Cross, and Wright, "Trial of Cannabidiol for Drug-Resistant Seizures," 699–700; Thiele et al., "Cannabidiol in Patients with Seizures Associated with Lennox-Gastaut Syndrome," 1085–96; Szaflarski et al., "Cannabidiol in Children and Adults with Treatment-Resistant Epilepsies," 1540–48; and Rosenberg et al., "Cannabinoids and Epilepsy," 747–68.

30. Schindler et al., "Migraine-Suppressing Effects of Psilocybin," 534–43.

31. Mayo Clinic Staff, "Inflammatory Bowel Disease (IBD)."
32. See Puckett, "Psychedelics, the Microbiome, and IBD," for a full discussion as Thompson and Szabo (2020) describe possible mechanisms. See also Thompson and Szabo, "Psychedelics as a Novel Approach to Treating Autoimmune Conditions," 45–54.
33. "Lyme Disease," Centers for Disease Control and Prevention.
34. Roberts, "How to Keep Ticks from Biting."
35. Kinderlehrer, "Treatment of Neuropsychiatric Lyme Disease," 109–15.
36. Personal correspondence with Jim Fadiman.
37. Masha, *Microdosing with Amanita muscaria,* 275.
38. Khosla, Patel, and Sharma, "Palliative Care in India," 149–54.
39. Downar and Lapenskie, "PSYCHED-PAL."
40. "NZ Trial," Radio New Zealand.
41. Founded by Rick Doblin, MAPS has spearheaded the introduction of psychedelic therapy in the United States and throughout the world.
42. See http://delospsyche.org.
43. "Hormones and PMDD," International Association for Premenstrual Disorders.
44. "PMDD in Young Adults," Newport Institute.
45. Quoted in Romaszkan, "ADHD and Premenstrual Dysphoric Disorder." Ally McHugh, a psychotherapist from the United Kingdom, is cofounder of the PMDD Collective, a team of mental health professionals focused on treating PMDD.
46. Eisenlohr-Moul et al., "Lifetime Self-Injurious Thoughts."
47. Tiranini and Nappi, "Understanding/Management of Premenstrual Dysphoric Disorder."
48. Williams, "Hailey's Microdosing Journey."
49. Personal correspondence with Jim.
50. Personal correspondence with Jim.
51. https://www.reddit.com/r/PsychedelicWomen.
52. "Premenstrual Syndrome," American College of Obstetricians and Gynecologists.
53. Haden, "Mark Haden from MAPS Canada."
54. Haden, Woods, and Paschall, "Psychedelics and Schizophrenia," 174–83.
55. Allen et al., "LSD Increases Sleep Duration."
56. u/Vintagecrawfish, "Psilocybin stroke recovery."
57. u/Vintagecrawfish.
58. u/nubpod23, "LSD or psilocybin microdosing good for stroke recovery?"
59. Oliver, "Psilocybin Microdosing and Stroke."
60. Oliver.
61. Masha, *Microdosing with Amanita Muscaria,* 70.
62. Hallifax, "Microdosing DMT to Treat Strokes."

63. "Stuttering," National Institute on Deafness and Other Communication Disorders.

64. Stamets, "How Paul Stamets STOPPED Stuttering."

65. "Traumatic Brain Injury," Johns Hopkins Medicine.

66. NFL Concussion Settlement website, https://www.nflconcussionsettlement.com /Reports_Statistics.aspx. See also *The Washington Post* report on the controversial administration of the settlement in Hobson, "The Concussion Files."

67. Multidisciplinary Association for Psychedelic Studies (MAPS), founded in 1986.

68. Mayo Clinic Staff, "Shingles."

6: Science and History

1. Interviewed by Lex Friedman, 2023.

2. Nutt, *Psychedelics,* 237.

3. Nutt.

4. Rootman et al., "Lower Levels of Anxiety and Depression."

5. Sharp and Bonnelle, "Tiny Doses, Big Samples."

6. Sharp and Bonnelle.

7. Rootman, "Findings from Microdose.me Study."

8. Rootman.

9. Rootman et al., "Psilocybin Microdosers."

10. Jay, "19th-Century Trippers."

11. Quoted in personal correspondence from Torsten Passie to James Fadiman, 2024.

12. Maslow, *The Psychology of Science.*

13. Jay, "19th-Century Trippers."

14. Jay.

15. Jay.

16. Quoted in "History of Citizen Science," UCL Library Services.

17. Hashkes, "Precise Definition of Microdosing Psychedelics Is Needed."

18. Wade, "Complexity of Your Brain Signals."

19. Polito, "Is Microdosing Just Placebo?"

20. Polito.

21. Nutt, *Psychedelics,* 243–45.

22. Murray, "New LSD Microdosing Research with Dana Harvey and Conor Murray."

23. Ackerman, "What Is Neuroplasticity?"

24. Calder and Hasler, "Psychedelic-Induced Neuroplasticity," 104–12.

25. Alcover and Mazo, "Plasticidad Cerebral y Hábito en William James."

26. James, "Habit."

27. Lieff, *Secret Language of Cells,* 93 et seq.

28. Dzyubenko and Hermann, "Role of Glia and Extracellular Matrix," 377–87.

29. Kargbo, "Psychedelic-Assisted Neuroplasticity," 133–35.

30. Huberman, "How Psilocybin Can Rewire Our Brain."

31. Calder and Hasler, "Psychedelic-Induced Neuroplasticity," 104–12.

32. Moliner et al., "Psychedelics Promote Plasticity," 1032–41.

33. Calder and Hasler, "Psychedelic-Induced Neuroplasticity," 104–12.

34. Martin, "Benefits of Microdosing."

35. Hirschfeld et al., "LSD-Induced Subjective Experiences," 1602–11.

36. Calder and Hasler, "Psychedelic-Induced Neuroplasticity," 104–12.

37. Huberman, "How Psilocybin Can Rewire Our Brain."

38. Aleksandrova and Phillips, "Neuroplasticity as a Convergent Mechanism," 929–42.

39. Friedman, "Psychedelics Open Your Brain."

40. Calder and Hasler, "Psychedelic-Induced Neuroplasticity," 104–12.

41. Huberman, "How Psilocybin Can Rewire Our Brain."

42. Pahwa, Goyal, and Jialal, "Chronic Inflammation."

43. Sohn, "Inflammaging."

44. Raz, "Transforming Psychedelics into Mainstream Medicines."

45. Thompson and Szabo, "Novel Approach," 45–54.

46. Nichols, "Anti-inflammatory Therapeutics."

47. Nichols.

48. Nichols.

49. Thomas, "Heart Health Risks of Microdosing."

50. Droogmans et al., "*3,4-Methylenedioxymethamphetamine* Abuse," 1442–45.

51. Hahn, "MDMA Toxicity."

52. Rouaud, Calder, and Hasler, "Risk of Cardiac Fibrosis and Valvulopathy."

53. Batra, "Homeopathy Continues to Gain Popularity."

54. "Homeopathy," National Center for Complementary and Integrative Health.

55. Doehring and Sundrum, "Efficacy of Homeopathy in Livestock."

56. Loudon, "Brief History of Homeopathy," 607–10.

57. Stannard, *American Holocaust*.

58. Celidwen et al., "Ethical Principles of Traditional Indigenous Medicine to Guide Western Psychedelic Research and Practice."

59. "María Sabina: Biography," Last.fm.

60. "María Sabina."

61. Brown and Brown, *The Psychedelic Gospels*.

62. Passie, *The Science of Microdosing Psychedelics*.

63. jdyf333, "I invented the word 'microdose.'"

64. jdyf333, "jdyf333: Overview."

65. jdyf333 "my 'MICRODOSE LSD' product insert."

66. jdyf333.

67. Leonard, "Hot New Business Trip."

68. Glatter, "Job Enhancer in Silicon Valley."
69. Solon, "Silicon Valley Workers."

7: Conclusions

1. Wilber, *Many Ways*, 4.

References

Ackerman, Courtney E. "What Is Neuroplasticity? A Psychologist Explains (+14 Tools)." Positive Psychology, July 25, 2018. https://positivepsychology.com/neuro plasticity.

Alcover, Carlos María, and Fernando Rodríguez Mazo. "Plasticidad Cerebral y Hábito en William James: Un Antecedente para la Neurociencia Social" [Brain Plasticity and Habit in William James: An Antecedent for Social Neuroscience]. *Psychologia Latina* 3, no. 1 (May 2012). http://dx.doi.org/10.5209/rev_PSLA .2012.v3.n1.38737.

Aleksandrova, Lily R., and Anthony G. Phillips. "Neuroplasticity as a Convergent Mechanism of Ketamine and Classical Psychedelics." *Trends in Pharmacological Sciences* 42, no. 11 (November 2021): 929–42. https://doi.org/10.1016/j.tips.2021.08.003.

All Things Amanita. https://allthingsamanita.com.

Allen, Nathan, Aron Jeremiah, Robin Murphy, Rachael Sumner, Anna Forsyth, Nicholas Hoeh, David B. Menkes, et al. "LSD Increases Sleep Duration the Night after Microdosing." *Translational Psychiatry* 14 (April 2024): 191. https://doi.org/10.1038 /s41398-024-02900-4.

Andersson, Martin, and Anette Kjellgren. "Twenty Percent Better with 20 Micrograms? A Qualitative Study of Psychedelic Microdosing Self-Rapports and Discussions on YouTube." *Harm Reduction Journal* 16 (November 2019): 63. https://doi.org/10.1186 /s12954-019-0333-3.

Anonymous. "The Secret to My Successful Career: Microdosing Magic Mushrooms." *The Times* (London), February 10, 2024. https://www.thetimes.co.uk/article/the-secret -to-my-successful-career-microdosing-magic-mushrooms-vnt6zr7x7.

"Assessing Your Weight." Centers for Disease Control and Prevention. US Department of Health and Human Services, June 3, 2022. https://www.cdc.gov/healthyweight /assessing/index.html.

Avi Esther, Natural Medicine Woman, www.aviesther.com.

Bansal, Narinder, Mohammed Hudda, Rupert A. Payne, Daniel J. Smith, David Kessler, and Nicola Wiles. "Antidepressant Use and Risk of Adverse Outcomes: Population-Based Cohort Study." *British Journal of Psychiatry Open* 8, no. 5 (September 2022): e164. https://doi.org/10.1192/bjo.2022.563.

Barba, Tommaso, Hannes Kettner, Caterina Radu, Joseph M. Peill, Leor Roseman, David J. Nutt, David Erritzoe, Robin Carhart-Harris, and Bruna Giribaldi. "Psychedelics and Sexual Functioning: A Mixed-Methods Study." *Scientific Reports* 14 (February 2024): 2181. https://doi.org/10.1038/s41598-023-49817-4.

Barnett, Brian S., Noah Wiles Sweat, and Peter S. Hendricks. "Case Report: Prolonged Amelioration of Mild Red-Green Color Vision Deficiency Following Psilocybin Mushroom Use." *Drug Science, Policy and Law* 9 (January–December 2023). https:// doi.org/10.1177/20503245231172536.

Batra, Mukesh. "Despite All Odds—Homeopathy Continues to Gain Popularity." *Voices* (blog). *Times of India,* July 20, 2022. https://timesofindia.indiatimes.com/blogs/voices /despite-all-odds-homeopathy-continues-to-gain-popularity.

Ben-Aharon, Avivit. "Celebrities Who Stutter." Great Speech, February 10, 2023. https:// greatspeech.com/celebrities-who-stutter.

"Benefits of Microdosing." Microdosing Institute. https://microdosinginstitute.com /microdosing-101/benefits.

Bezos, Jeff. "Jeff Bezos: Amazon and Blue Origin | Lex Fridman Podcast #405." Interview by Lex Fridman. Uploaded December 14, 2023. YouTube video, 2:11:31. https:// www.youtube.com/watch?v=DcWqzZ3I2cY.

"Bipolar Disorder." National Institute of Mental Health. US Department of Health and Human Services, February 2024. https://www.nimh.nih.gov/health/topics/bipolar -disorder.

Blesching, Uwe. *The Cannabis Health Index: Combining the Science of Medical Marijuana with Mindfulness Techniques to Heal 100 Chronic Symptoms and Diseases.* Berkeley, CA: North Atlantic Books, 2015.

Bonnelle, Valerie, Will J. Smith, Natasha L. Mason, Mauro Cavarra, Pamela Kryskow, Kim P. C. Kuypers, Johannes G. Ramaekers, and Amanda Feilding. "Analgesic Potential of Macrodoses and Microdoses of Classic Psychedelics in Chronic Pain Sufferers: A Population Survey." *British Journal of Pain* 16, no. 6 (December 2022): 619–31. https:// doi.org/10.1177/20494637221114962.

Bornemann, Joel. "The Viability of Microdosing Psychedelics as a Strategy to Enhance Cognition and Well-Being: An Early Review." *Journal of Psychoactive Drugs* 52, no. 4 (September–October 2020): 300–308. https://doi.org/10.1080/02791072.2020 .1761573.

Braman, Sidney S. "The Global Burden of Asthma." In "Decreasing the Global Burden of Asthma." *Chest* 130, no. 1 Suppl. (July 2006): 4S–12S. https://doi.org/10.1378 /chest.130.1_suppl.4S.

Bramlage, Adam. Flow State Micro. https://www.flowstatemicro.com.

Brown, Jerry B., and Julie M. Brown. *The Psychedelic Gospels: The Secret History of Hallucinogens in Christianity.* Rochester, VT: Park Street Press, 2016.

Brumback, T., N. Castro, J. Jacobus, and S. Tapert. "Effects of Marijuana Use on Brain Structure and Function: Neuroimaging Findings from a Neurodevelopmental Perspective." *International Review of Neurobiology* 129 (2016): 33–65. https://doi.org /10.1016/bs.irn.2016.06.004.

"Busting Protocol—The Dosing Method." Clusterbusters, April 25, 2023. https:// clusterbusters.org/resource/the-dosing-method.

Calder, Abigail E., and Gregor Hasler. "Towards an Understanding of Psychedelic-Induced Neuroplasticity." *Neuropsychopharmacology* 48, no. 1 (January 2023): 104–12. https://doi.org/10.1038/s41386-022-01389-z.

"Can You Use *Amanita muscaria* to Help Relieve Pain and Anxiety?" *Clinton Courier,* September 26, 2023. https://www.theclintoncourier.net/2023/09/26/can-you-use -amanita-muscaria-to-help-relieve-pain-and-anxiety.

Celidwen, Yuria, Nicole Redvers, Cicilia Githaiga, Janeth Calambás, Karen Añaños, Miguel Evanjuanoy Chindoy, Riccardo Vitale, et al. "Ethical Principles of Traditional Indigenous Medicine to Guide Western Psychedelic Research and Practice." *Personal View* 18 (February 2023): 100410. https://doi.org/10.1016/j.lana.2022 .100410.

Chan, Chi Chao, Martin Fishman, and Peter R. Egbert. "Multiple Ocular Anomalies Associated with Maternal LSD Ingestion." *Archives of Ophthalmology* 96, no. 2 (February 1978): 282–84. https://doi.org/10.1001/archopht.1978.03910050150009.

"Chronic Pain." Johns Hopkins Medicine. https://www.hopkinsmedicine.org/health /conditions-and-diseases/chronic-pain.

Cooper, Ziva D., Maria A. Sullivan, Suzanne K. Vosburg, Jeanne M. Manubay, Margaret Haney, Richard W. Foltin, Suzette M. Evans, William J. Kowalczyk, Phillip A. Saccone, and Sandra D. Comer. "Effects of Repeated Oxycodone Administration on Its Analgesic and Subjective Effects in Normal, Healthy Volunteers." *Behavioural Pharmacology* 23, no. 3 (June 2012): 271–79. https://doi.org/10.1097/FBP .0b013e3283536d6f.

Cormier, Zoe. "No Link Found Between Psychedelics and Psychosis." *Scientific American,* March 4, 2015. https://www.scientificamerican.com/article/no-link-found-between -psychedelics-and-psychosis1.

Danielson, Melissa L., Michele K. Bohm, Kimberly Newsome, Angelika H. Claussen, Jennifer W. Kaminski, Scott D. Grosse, Lila Siwakoti, Aziza Arifkhanova, Rebecca H. Bitsko, and Lara R. Robinson. "Trends in Stimulant Prescription Fills Among Commercially Insured Children and Adults—United States, 2016–2021." *Morbidity and Mortality Weekly Report* 72, no. 13 (March 31, 2023): 327–32. https://doi.org/10.15585/mmwr.mm7213a1.

Davis, Erik. *Blotter: The Untold Story of an Acid Medium.* Cambridge, MA: MIT Press, 2024.

Devinsky, Orrin, J. Helen Cross, and Stephen Wright. "Trial of Cannabidiol for Drug-Resistant Seizures in the Dravet Syndrome." *New England Journal of Medicine* 377, no. 7 (August 2017): 699–700. https://doi.org/10.1056/NEJMc1708349.

deVos, Corey, and Ryan Oelke. "Inhabit: Your Wokeness." Inhabit. Integral Life, May 4, 2021. Video, 1:25:52. https://integrallife.com/inhabit-your-wokeness.

Doehring, C., and A. Sundrum. "Efficacy of Homeopathy in Livestock According to Peer-Reviewed Publications from 1981 to 2014." *Veterinary Record* 179, no. 24 (December 2016): 628. https://doi.org/10.1136/vr.103779.

Dölen, Gül. "Psychedelics Unlock Learning Windows in the Brain." Neuroscience News, June 14, 2023. https://neurosciencenews.com/psychedelics-social-learning-23466.

Downar, James, and Julie Lapenskie. "PSilocybin for psYCHological and Existential Distress in PALliative Care (PSYCHED-PAL): A Multi-Site, Open-Label, Single Arm Phase I/II Proof-of-Concept, Dose-Finding, and Feasibility Clinical Trial." Ongoing study. Last updated January 14, 2024. https://clinicaltrials.gov/study/NCT04754061.

Droogmans, Steven, Bernard Cosyns, Hugo D'haenen, Edwin Creeten, Caroline Weytjens, Philippe R. Franken, Benjamin Scott, et al. "Possible Association Between *3,4-Methylenedioxymethamphetamine* Abuse and Valvular Heart Disease." *American Journal of Cardiology* 100, no. 9 (November 2007): 1442–45. https://doi.org/10.1016/j.amjcard.2007.06.045.

"Drug Scheduling." United States Drug Enforcement Administration. US Department of Justice, July 10, 2018. https://www.dea.gov/drug-information/drug-scheduling.

Ducharme, Jamie. "The Latest Promising Long COVID Treatment? Psychedelic Drugs." *Time,* April 17, 2023. https://time.com/6271806/psychedelics-long-covid-treatment.

———. "Long COVID Recovery Remains Rare. Doctors Are Struggling to Understand Why." *Time,* August 29, 2023. https://time.com/6309054/long-covid-recovery-rare.

———. "What's Driving the Demand for ADHD Drugs Like Adderall." *Time,* April 12, 2023. https://time.com/6271049/adhd-diagnoses-rising.

———. "Why So Many Long COVID Patients Are Reporting Suicidal Thoughts." *Time,* June 13, 2022. https://time.com/6186429/suicide-long-covid.

Dysphoric Project. https://DysphoricProject.org.

Dzyubenko, Egor, and Dirk M. Hermann. "Role of Glia and Extracellular Matrix in Controlling Neuroplasticity in the Central Nervous System." *Seminars in Immunopathology* 45, no. 3 (May 2023): 377–87. https://doi.org/10.1007/s00281-023-00989-1.

"Eating Disorder Statistics." South Carolina Department of Mental Health. https://www.state.sc.us/dmh/anorexia/statistics.htm.

"Eating Disorders." National Institute of Mental Health. US Department of Health and Human Services, January 2024. https://www.nimh.nih.gov/health/topics/eating-disorders.

Ehrlichman, John. "Drug War Confessional." Vera Institute of Justice. https://www.vera.org/reimagining-prison-webumentary/the-past-is-never-dead/drug-war-confessional.

Eisenlohr-Moul, Tory, Madeline Divine, Katja Schmalenberger, Laura Murphy, Brett Buchert, Melissa Wagner-Schuman, Alyssa Kania, et al. "Prevalence of Lifetime Self-Injurious Thoughts and Behaviors in a Global Sample of 599 Patients Reporting Prospectively Confirmed Diagnosis with Premenstrual Dysphoric Disorder." *BMC Psychiatry* 22, no. 1 (March 2022): 199. https://doi.org/10.1186/s12888-022-03851-0.

Eubanks, Chris. "My Experience Microdosing to Learn a Language." Medium, November 10, 2022. https://eubanks.medium.com/my-experience-microdosing-to-learn-a-language-8f1c7ba7d801 (post removed).

"Experience with micro-dosing psilocybin. Bipolar folks only please." r/Microdosing. Reddit, July 25, 2022. https://www.reddit.com/r/microdosing/comments/w7vsxe/experience_with_microdosing_psilocybin_bipolar. The account that originated this thread has since been deleted.

Fadiman, James. *The Psychedelic Explorer's Guide: Safe, Therapeutic, and Sacred Journeys.* Rochester, VT: Park Street Press, 2011.

Fadiman, James, and Jordan Gruber. *Your Symphony of Selves: Discover and Understand More of Who We Are.* Rochester, VT: Park Street Press, 2020.

Fadiman, James, and Sophia Korb. "Might Microdosing Psychedelics Be Safe and Beneficial? An Initial Exploration." *Journal of Psychoactive Drugs* 51, no. 2 (April–June 2019): 118–22. https://doi.org/10.1080/02791072.2019.1593561.

Fadiman, James, and Andrew Kornfeld. "Psychedelic-Induced Experiences." Chap. 19 in *The Wiley Blackwell Handbook of Transpersonal Psychology,* edited by Harris L. Friedman and Glenn Hartelius, 352–66. Chichester, UK: John Wiley and Sons, 2013. https://doi.org/10.1002/9781118591277.ch19.

Feeney, Kevin M., ed. *Fly Agaric: A Compendium of History, Pharmacology, Mythology, and Exploration.* Ellensburg, WA: Fly Agaric Press, 2020.

Fink, Erica. "When Silicon Valley Takes LSD." CNN Money, January 25, 2015. https://money.cnn.com/2015/01/25/technology/lsd-psychedelics-silicon-valley.

Finney, Ali. "Is Smoking Weed Bad for Your Heart?" *Self,* February 26, 2024. https://self.com/story/weed-cannabis-heart-health.

Fried, Eiko I. "The 52 Symptoms of Major Depression: Lack of Content Overlap Among Seven Common Depression Scales." *Journal of Affective Disorders* 208 (January 2017): 191–97. https://doi.org/10.1016/j.jad.2016.10.019.

Friedman, Richard A. "Psychedelics Open Your Brain. You Might Not Like What Falls In." *The Atlantic,* February 1, 2023. https://www.theatlantic.com/health/archive/2023/02/psychedelic-drug-therapy-effects-brain-neuroplasticity/672910.

Garcia-Romeu, Albert, Frederick S. Barrett, Theresa M. Carbonaro, Matthew W. Johnson, and Roland R. Griffiths. "Optimal Dosing for Psilocybin Pharmacotherapy: Considering Weight-Adjusted and Fixed Dosing Approaches." *Journal of Psychopharmacology* 35, no. 4 (April 2021): 353–61. https://doi.org/10.1177/0269881121991822.

Ghaemi, Nassir. "Has the Serotonin Hypothesis Been Debunked?" *Mood Swings* (blog). *Psychology Today*, October 1, 2022. https://www.psychologytoday.com/us/blog/mood-swings/202210/has-the-serotonin-hypothesis-been-debunked.

Glatter, Robert. "LSD Microdosing: The New Job Enhancer in Silicon Valley and Beyond?" *Forbes,* November 27, 2015. https://www.forbes.com/sites/robertglatter/2015/11/27/lsd-microdosing-the-new-job-enhancer-in-silicon-valley-and-beyond.

Grabski, Isabelle. "Can Calorie Restriction Extend Your Lifespan?" *Science in the News* (blog). Harvard Graduate School of the Arts and Sciences, August 2, 2020. https://sitn.hms.harvard.edu/flash/2020/can-microdosing-psychedelics-improve-your-mental-health.

———. "Can Microdosing Psychedelics Improve Your Mental Health?" *Science in the News* (blog). Harvard Graduate School of the Arts and Sciences, December 18, 2020. https://sitn.hms.harvard.edu/flash/2020/can-microdosing-psychedelics-improve-your-mental-health.

Griffiths, R. R., W. A. Richards, U. McCann, and R. Jesse. "Psilocybin Can Occasion Mystical-Type Experiences Having Substantial and Sustained Personal Meaning and Spiritual Significance." *Psychopharmacology* 187, no. 3 (August 2006): 268–83.

"A Guide to Microdosing *Banisteriopsis caapi* Vine." Microdosing Institute. https://microdosinginstitute.com/microdosing-101/substances/microdosing-b-caapi-vine.

Gupta, Sarah. "Bipolar 1 vs. 2: Understanding the Difference Between These Mental Health Conditions." GoodRX Health, August 30, 2022. https://www.goodrx.com/conditions/bipolar-disorder/bipolar-1-vs-2-differences.

Haden, Mark. "Mark Haden from MAPS Canada." Interview by David McNee. *The Psychedelic Suitcase* (podcast), October 8, 2019. https://www.listennotes.com/podcasts/the-psychedelic/003-mark-haden-from-maps-_8t12QCvmni/?t=1186#1186.

Haden, Mark, Birgitta Anne Woods, and Sarah A. Paschall. "Psychedelics and Schizophrenia: A Mystery in History." *Journal of Psychedelic Studies* 7, no. 3 (December 2023): 174–83. https://doi.org/10.1556/2054.2023.00277.

Hahn, In-Hei. "MDMA Toxicity." Medscape. WebMD, August 21, 2023. https://emedicine.medscape.com/article/821572-overview.

Haichin, Michael. "The Interdisciplinary Annotated Psychedelic Research Bibliography of 2023." Psychedelic Alpha. https://psychedelicalpha.com/news/2023-annotated-interdisciplinary-psychedelics-bibliography. This annotated bibliography contains "over 500 notable psychedelics-related publications from 2023," most of which are not about microdosing.

Haigney, Zach. "The Curious Connection Between Psychedelics and Longevity." *The Trip Report by Beckley Waves* (blog), September 17, 2021. https://www.thetripreport.com /p/the-curious-connection-between-psychedelics.

Haijen, Eline C. H. M., Petra P. M. Hurks, and Kim P. C. Kuypers. "Microdosing with Psychedelics to Self-Medicate for ADHD Symptoms in Adults: A Prospective Naturalistic Study." *Neuroscience Applied* 1 (2022): 101012. https://doi.org/10.1016/j.nsa .2022.101012.

———. "Trait Mindfulness and Personality Characteristics in a Microdosing ADHD Sample: A Naturalistic Prospective Survey Study." *Frontiers in Psychiatry* 14 (October 2023): 1233585. https://doi.org/10.3389/fpsyt.2023.1233585.

Hallifax, James. "Microdosing DMT to Treat Strokes: Not as Trippy as It Sounds." Microdose. MD Media, January 18, 2023. https://microdose.buzz/news/microdosing -dmt-to-treat-stokes-not-as-trippy-as-it-sounds.

"Hallucinations and Hearing Voices." National Health Service (UK), February 15, 2022. https://www.nhs.uk/mental-health/feelings-symptoms-behaviours/feelings-and -symptoms/hallucinations-hearing-voices.

Hartogsohn, Ido. "Constructing Drug Effects: A History of Set and Setting." *Drug Science Policy and Law* 3, no. 1 (January 2017). https://doi.org/10.1177/2050324516683325.

Hatton, Ian A., Eric D. Galbraith, Nono S. C. Merleau, Teemu P. Miettinen, Benjamin McDonald Smith, and Jeffery A. Shander. "The Human Cell Count and Size Distribution." *Proceedings of the National Academy of Sciences* 120, no. 39 (September 2023): e2303077120. https://doi.org/10.1073/pnas.2303077120.

Hashkes, Sarah. "A Precise Definition of Microdosing Psychedelics Is Needed to Promote Equitable Regulation." *Bill of Health* (blog). Petrie-Flom Center. Harvard Law School, April 5, 2022. https://blog.petrieflom.law.harvard.edu/2022/04/05 /microdosing-psychedelics-definition.

Heifets, Boris D., and David E. Olson. "Therapeutic Mechanisms of Psychedelics and Entactogens." *Neuropsychopharmacology* 49, no. 1 (January 2024): 104–18. https://doi .org/10.1038/s41386-023-01666-5.

Hicks, Alexandra. "Top Mescaline Producing Cacti from Around the World." *Cannadelics Sunday Edition* (newsletter), September 15, 2023. https://cannadelics.com/2023/09 /15/top-mescaline-producing-cacti-from-around-the-world.

Hirschfeld, Tim, Johanna Prugger, Tomislav Majić, and Timo T. Schmidt. "Dose-Response Relationships of LSD-Induced Subjective Experiences in Humans." *Neuropsychopharmacology* 48, no. 11 (October 2023): 1602–11. https://doi.org/10.1038 /s41386-023-01588-2.

"History of Citizen Science." UCL Library Services. University College London. https:// www.ucl.ac.uk/library/open-science-research-support/open-science/citizen-science /history-citizen-science.

"History of the Royal Society." Royal Society. https://royalsociety.org/about-us/history.

Hobson, Will. "The Concussion Files." *Washington Post,* January 31, 2024. https://www.washingtonpost.com/sports/interactive/2024/nfl-concussion-settlement.

Hofmann, Albert, Rick Doblin, Charles Grob, John Halpern, Michael Mithoefer, and Andrew Sewell. "Albert Hofmann Speaks." *Entheogen Review* 14, no. 1 (September 2005): 83–93.

"Homeopathy: What You Need to Know." National Center for Complementary and Integrative Health. US Department of Health and Human Services, April 2021. https://www.nccih.nih.gov/health/homeopathy.

"Hormones and PMDD." International Association for Premenstrual Disorders, April 23, 2019. https://iapmd.org/hormones-and-pmd.

"How Does Social Connectedness Affect Health?" Centers for Disease Control and Prevention. US Department of Health and Human Services, March 30, 2023. https://www.cdc.gov/emotional-wellbeing/social-connectedness/affect-health.htm.

Huberman, Andrew. "How Psilocybin Can Rewire Our Brain, Its Therapeutic Benefits and Its Risks." Huberman Lab. Scicomm Media, May 7, 2023. Video, 2:09:02. https://www.hubermanlab.com/episode/how-psilocybin-can-rewire-our-brain-its-therapeutic-benefits-and-its-risks.

Hutten, Nadia R. P. W., Natasha L. Mason, Patrick C. Dolder, and Kim P. C. Kuypers. "Self-Rated Effectiveness of Microdosing with Psychedelics for Mental and Physical Health Problems Among Microdosers." *Frontiers in Psychiatry* 10 (September 2019): 672. https://doi.org/10.3389/fpsyt.2019.00672.

Huxley, Aldous. *The Doors of Perception.* New York: Harper and Row, 1954.

Inbar, Kineret, Liran A. Levi, and Yonatan M. Kupchik. "Cocaine Induces Input and Cell-Type-Specific Synaptic Plasticity in Ventral Pallidum-Projecting Nucleus Accumbens Medium Spiny Neurons." *Neuropsychopharmacology* 47, no. 8 (July 2022): 1461–72. https://doi.org/10.1038/s41386-022-01285-6.

"Investigation of Illnesses: Diamond Shruumz-Brand Chocolate Bars, Cones, & Gummies (June 2024)." United States Food and Drug Administration, July 23, 2024. https://www.fda.gov/food/outbreaks-foodborne-illness/investigation-illnesses-diamond-shruumz-brand-chocolate-bars-cones-gummies-june-2024.

Ironwood, Patrick, curator of *The Psychedelic Universe Club* on Clubhouse, https://brewstersociety.com/artist/patrick-ironwood-2.

Isra. "What Is Lemon Tekking?" The Level, May 30, 2023. https://thelevel.org.nz/news-and-stories/lemon-tekking.

Jaeger, Kyle. "DEA Confirms That Psychedelic Mushroom Spores Are Federally Legal Prior to Germination." Marijuana Moment, January 4, 2024. https://www.marijuanamoment.net/dea-confirms-that-psychedelic-mushroom-spores-are-federally-legal-prior-to-germination.

Jakobsen, Janus Christian, Christian Gluud, and Irving Kirsch. "Should Antidepressants Be Used for Major Depressive Disorder?" *BMJ Evidence-Based Medicine* 25, no. 4 (August 2020): 130–36. https://doi.org/10.1136/bmjebm-2019-111238.

James, William. "Habit." Chap. 4 in *The Principles of Psychology*. New York: Henry Holt, 1890. https://psychclassics.yorku.ca/James/Principles/prin4.htm.

Jay, Mike. "The 19th-Century Trippers Who Probed the Mind." *Nautilus,* May 10, 2023. https://nautil.us/the-19th-century-trippers-who-probed-the-mind-303265.

———. *Psychonauts: Drugs and the Making of the Modern Mind*. New Haven: Yale University Press, 2023.

Jewell, Tim. "What's the Difference Between Asperger's and Autism?" Healthline, April 16, 2020. https://www.healthline.com/health/aspergers-vs-autism.

jdyf333. "I invented the word 'microdose.'" Flickr, June 8, 2020. https://www.flickr.com/photos/jdyf333/51798043923.

———. "My 'MICRODOSE LSD' product insert (from early 1988)." Flickr, June 7, 2020. https://www.flickr.com/photos/jdyf333/2075297284.

Kargbo, Robert B. "Psychedelic-Assisted Neuroplasticity for the Treatment of Mental Health Disorders." *ACS Medicinal Chemistry Letters* 14, no. 2 (January 2023): 133–35. https://doi.org/10.1021/acsmedchemlett.2c00546.

Kelly, John R., Gerard Clarke, Andrew Harkin, Sinead C. Corr, Stephen Galvin, Vishnu Pradeep, John F. Cryan, Veronica O'Keane, and Timothy G. Dinan. "Seeking the Psilocybiome: Psychedelics Meet the Microbiota-Gut-Brain Axis." *International Journal of Clinical and Health Psychology* 23, no. 2 (April–June 2023): 100349. https://doi.org/10.1016/j.ijchp.2022.100349.

Kempner, Joanna. *Psychedelic Outlaws: The Movement Revolutionizing Modern Medicine*. New York: Hachette, 2024.

Kinderlehrer, Daniel A. "The Effectiveness of Microdosed Psilocybin in the Treatment of Neuropsychiatric Lyme Disease: A Case Study." *International Medical Case Reports Journal* 16 (March 2023): 109–15. https://doi.org/10.2147/IMCRJ.S395342.

Khosla, Divya, Firuza D. Patel, and Suresh C. Sharma. "Palliative Care in India: Current Progress and Future Needs." *Indian Journal of Palliative Care* 18, no. 3 (September 2012): 149–54. https://doi.org/10.4103/0973-1075.105683.

Kirsch, Irving. *The Emperor's New Drugs: Exploding the Antidepressant Myth*. New York: Basic Books, 2010.

Klayman, Alison, dir. *Take Your Pills*. Brooklyn: Motto Pictures and Netflix Studios, 2018. https://www.netflix.com/title/80117831.

Kliegman, Julie. "What Do Athletes Get from Ayahuasca, Mushrooms and Ecstasy?" Daily Cover. *Sports Illustrated,* August 12, 2022. https://www.si.com/more-sports/2022/08/12/psychedelics-sports-aaron-rodgers-daily-cover.

Latifi, Fortesa. "Are Mushrooms the Social Drug of 2024? An Investigation." Refinery29.

VICE Media Group, December 20, 2023. https://www.refinery29.com/en-us /microdosing-mushrooms-psilocybin-trend-explained.

Lang, Thomas A., and Donna F. Stroup. "Who Knew? The Misleading Specificity of 'Double-Blind' and What to Do About It." *Trials* 21 (August 2020): 697. https://doi .org/10.1186/s13063-020-04607-5.

Lattin, Don. *God on Psychedelics: Tripping Across the Rubble of Old-Time Religion.* Hannacroix, NY: Apocryphile Press, 2023.

Leonard, Andrew. "How LSD Microdosing Became the Hot New Business Trip." *Rolling Stone,* November 20, 2015. https://www.rollingstone.com/culture/culture-news/how -lsd-microdosing-became-the-hot-new-business-trip-64961.

Lewis-Healy, Evan. "Why Psychedelics Could Eventually Treat Asthma." Psychedelic Spotlight. PSYC Media, July 12, 2021. https://psychedelicspotlight.com/psychedelics -could-treat-asthma.

Lieber, Chavie. "The Working Woman's Newest Life Hack: Magic Mushrooms." *Wall Street Journal,* February 4, 2024. https://www.wsj.com/style/microdosing-mushrooms -psilocybin-trend-women-f8d28b72.

Lieff, Jon. *The Secret Language of Cells: What Biological Conversations Tell Us About the Brain–Body Connection, the Future of Medicine, and Life Itself.* Dallas: BenBella Books, 2020.

Long, Sally Y. "Does LSD Induce Chromosomal Damage and Malformations? A Review of the Literature." *Teratology* 6, no. 1 (August 1972): 75–90. https://doi.org/10.1002 /tera.1420060110.

Loudon, Irvine. "A Brief History of Homeopathy." *Journal of the Royal Society of Medicine* 99, no. 12 (December 2006): 607–10. https://doi.org/10.1258%2Fjrsm.99 .12.607.

Love, Shayla. "'Long-Lost Best Friends': The Longevity Movement Finds Psychedelics." *The Guardian,* December 8, 2023. https://www.theguardian.com/wellness/2023/dec /08/longevity-psychedelics-mental-health-ageing.

"Lyme Disease." Centers for Disease Control and Prevention. US Department of Health and Human Services, January 19, 2022. https://cdc.gov/lyme/index.html.

Mama de la Myco. https://www.mushwomb.love.

Mama de la Myco. *Things We Learned from Mushroom Mothers.* Mothers of the Mushroom. https://www.canva.com/design/DAF3VO4NsFo/AXiW1suECqmfPnk3OOzVyA /view#1.

Manchester, William. *A World Lit Only by Fire: The Medieval Mind and the Renaissance; Portrait of an Age.* Boston: Little, Brown, 1992.

"María Sabina: Biography." Last.fm. https://www.last.fm/music/Mar%C3%ADa+Sabina /+wiki.

Markoff, John. *What the Dormouse Said: How the Sixties Counterculture Shaped the Personal Computer Industry.* New York: Viking, 2005.

Marks, Mason, I. Glenn Cohen, Jonathan Perez-Reyzin, and David Angelatos. "Microdosing Psychedelics Under Local, State, and Federal Law." *Boston University Law Review* 103, no. 2 (October 2023): 573–641. https://www.bu.edu/bulawreview/files/2023/10/MARKS.pdf.

Marlan, Dustin. "What Macrodosing Can Learn from Microdosing." *Bill of Health* (blog). Harvard Law School, April 6, 2022. https://blog.petrieflom.law.harvard.edu/2022/04/06/what-macrodosing-can-learn-from-microdosing.

Martin, Kelly. "What Are the Benefits of Microdosing?" Goop, August 2, 2022. https://goop.com/wellness/health/microdosing-psychedelics.

Marx, Danae. "Mushroom Extract Outperforms Synthetic Psilocybin in Psychiatric Therapy." Neuroscience News, March 12, 2024. https://neurosciencenews.com/psilocybin-mental-health-25739.

Masha, Baba. *Microdosing with Amanita Muscaria: Creativity, Healing, and Recovery with the Sacred Mushroom.* Rochester, VT: Park Street Press, 2022.

Maslow, Abraham H. *The Psychology of Science.* New York: Harper and Row, 1966.

Mayo Clinic Staff. "Inflammatory Bowel Disease (IBD)." Mayo Foundation for Medical Education and Research, September 3, 2022. https://www.mayoclinic.org/diseases-conditions/inflammatory-bowel-disease/diagnosis-treatment/drc-20353320.

———. "Shingles." Mayo Foundation for Medical Education and Research, August 20, 2022. https://www.mayoclinic.org/diseases-conditions/shingles/symptoms-causes/syc-20353054.

McConchie, James. Haight Street Shroom Shoppe, www.haightshroomshop.com.

McElory, Connor. "How Strong Is the Average Magic Mushroom?" Tripsitter, January 16, 2024. https://tripsitter.com/magic-mushrooms/average-potency.

McKenna, Dennis. "Joe Rogan on Micro-dosing Psilocybin." Interview by Joe Rogan. JRE Clips. Uploaded April 18, 2017. YouTube video, 7:21. https://www.youtube.com/watch?v=pUWaZ_wxhhg.

McKenna, Dennis, and Terence McKenna [O. T. Oss and O. N. Oeric, pseud.]. *Psilocybin: Magic Mushroom Grower's Guide.* Berkeley, CA: And/Or Press, 1976.

"Microdosing." Wikipedia. Wikimedia Foundation. https://en.wikipedia.org/wiki/Microdosing.

"Microdosing Psilocybin with Cacao." Pure Kakaw. https://purekakaw.com/pages/microdosing-psilocybin-with-cacao.

"Microdosing While Breastfeeding: How Safe Is It?" Microdosing Institute, May 9, 2022. https://microdosinginstitute.com/health/microdosing-mushrooms-while-breastfeeding-how-safe-is-it.

Microhuasca. https://www.microhuasca.com.

Microhuasca Institute. "Ayahuasca Microdosing: Findings, part 2." In *Program of Introduction to the Use of Microdoses of Ayahuasca.* Peru: Microhuasca Institute (2021).

Miller, Jessica. "Effects of Porn Addiction." AddictionHelp.com, March 25, 2024. https://www.addictionhelp.com/porn/effects.

MindBio Therapeutics. "MindBio Announces Sustained Antidepressant Response 3-Months

Post Treatment in Microdosing Depression Clinical Trials." News release, August 19, 2024. https://www.accesswire.com/903323/mindbio-announces-sustained-antidepressant-response-3-months-post-treatment-in-microdosing-depression-clinical-trials.

Moliner, Rafael, Mykhailo Girych, Cecilia A. Brunello, Vera Kovaleva, Caroline Biojone, Giray Enkavi, Lina Antenucci, et al. "Psychedelics Promote Plasticity by Directly Binding to BDNF Receptor TrkB." *Nature Neuroscience* 26, no. 6 (June 2023): 1032–41. https://doi.org/10.1038/s41593-023-01316-5.

Moncrieff, Joanna, and Mark Horowitz. "Analysis: Depression Is Probably Not Caused by a Chemical Imbalance in the Brain—New Study." The Conversation. UCL News. University College London, July 20, 2022. https://www.ucl.ac.uk/news/2022/jul/analysis-depression-probably-not-caused-chemical-imbalance-brain-new-study.

Muraresku, Brian C. *The Immortality Key: The Secret History of the Religion with No Name.* New York: St. Martin's Press, 2020.

Murray, Conor. "Microdosing Revealed: Boost Your Creativity and Happiness." Training video. Flow State Ventures, 2024. MP4 video.

Murray, Conor. "New LSD Microdosing Research with Dana Harvey and Conor Murray." Interview by Dana Harvey. *Psychedelic Revelations Podcast,* April 23, 2024. MP3 Audio, 1:36:19. https://podcasters.spotify.com/pod/show/psychedelic-revelations/episodes/New-LSD-Microdosing-Research-with-Dana-Harvey-and-Conor-Murray-e2ipmcd.

Murray, Conor H., Joel Frohlich, Connor J. Haggarty, Ilaria Tare, Royce Lee, and Harriet de Wit. "Neural Complexity Is Increased After Low Doses of LSD, but Not Moderate to High Doses of Oral THC or Methamphetamine." *Neuropsychopharmacology.* Published ahead of print, January 29, 2024. https://doi.org/10.1038/s41386-024-01809-2.

Myer, Marc. "Best Life: Adults Are the Biggest Consumers of Adderall Now." Interview by Ivanhoe Newswire. Action News 5. Gray Television, July 12, 2021. https://www.actionnews5.com/2021/07/12/best-life-adults-are-biggest-consumers-adderall-now.

Neiloufar Family, Emeline L. Maillet, Luke T. J. Williams, Erwin Krediet, Robin L. Carhart-Harris, Tim M. Williams, Charles D. Nichols, Daniel J. Goble, and Shlomi Raz. "Safety, Tolerability, Pharmacokinetics, and Pharmacodynamics of Low Dose Lysergic Acid Diethylamide (LSD) in Healthy Older Volunteers." *Psychopharmacology* 237, no. 3 (March 2020): 841–53. https://doi.org/10.1007/s00213-019-05417-7.

Neiloufar Family, David Vinson, Gabriella Vigliocco, Mendel Kaelen, Mark Bolstridge, David J. Nutt, and Robin L. Carhart-Harris. "Semantic Activation in LSD: Evidence from Picture Naming." *Language, Cognition and Neuroscience* 31, no. 10 (2016): 1320–27. https://doi.org/10.1080/23273798.2016.1217030.

Nichols, Charles D. "Eleusis Sheds Light on Psychedelics That Relieve Asthma in Rats with No Mental Effects." Interview by Arlene Weintraub. Fierce Biotech. Questex, August 13, 2020. https://www.fiercebiotech.com/research/eleusis-sheds-light-psychedelics-relieve-asthma-rats-no-mental-effects.

————. "Psychedelics as Potent Anti-inflammatory Therapeutics." *Neuropharmacology* 219 (November 2022): 109232. https://doi.org/10.1016/j.neuropharm.2022.109232.

Nierenberg, Andrew A., Bruno Agustini, Ole Köhler-Forsberg, Cristina Cusin, Douglas Katz, Louisa G. Sylvia, Amy Peters, and Michael Berk. "Diagnosis and Treatment of Bipolar Disorder: A Review." *JAMA* 330, no. 14 (October 2023): 1370–80. https://doi.org/10.1001/jama.2023.18588.

"No Evidence That Depression Is Caused by Low Serotonin Levels, Finds Comprehensive Review." UCL News. University College London, July 20, 2022. https://www.ucl.ac.uk/news/2022/jul/no-evidence-depression-caused-low-serotonin-levels-finds-comprehensive-review.

"Number of People Taking ADHD Drugs in the United States." Citizens Commission on Human Rights International, April 2018. https://www.cchrint.org/psychiatric-drugs/stimulantsideeffects/people-taking-adhd-drugs.

Nutt, David. *Psychedelics: The Revolutionary Drugs That Could Change Your Life—A Guide from the Expert.* London: Hodder and Stoughton, 2023.

"NZ Trial Explores Combining LSD with Therapy." Radio New Zealand, July 16, 2024. https://www.rnz.co.nz/news/national/522324/nz-trial-explores-combining-lsd-with-therapy.

Oliver, Dax. "Psilocybin Microdosing and Stroke: A Diary." Invisible Illness. Medium, February 20, 2020. https://medium.com/invisible-illness/psilocybin-microdosing-and-stroke-a-diary-7e5e7d4150f4.

Ona, Genís, and José Carlos Bouso. "Potential Safety, Benefits, and Influence of the Placebo Effect in Microdosing Psychedelic Drugs: A Systematic Review." *Neuroscience & Behavioral Reviews* 119 (December 2020): 194–203. https://doi.org/10.1016/j.neubiorev.2020.09.035.

Orsini, Aaron Paul. *Autism on Acid: How LSD Helped Me Understand, Navigate, Alter and Appreciate My Autistic Perceptions.* Self-published, 2020.

Pahwa, Roma, Amandeep Goyal, and Ishwarlal Jialal. "Chronic Inflammation." Treasure Island, FL: StatPearls Publishing, 2024. https://www.ncbi.nlm.nih.gov/books/NBK493173.

"Pain." MedlinePlus. National Library of Medicine, August 10, 2018. https://medlineplus.gov/pain.html.

Passie, Torsten. *The Science of Microdosing Psychedelics.* London: Psychedelic Press, 2019.

Petrilli, Kat, Shelan Ofori, Lindsey Hines, Gemma Taylor, Sally Adams, and Tom P. Freeman. "Association of Cannabis Potency with Mental Ill Health and Addiction: A Systematic Review." *Lancet* 9, no. 9 (September 2022): 736–50. https://doi.org/10.1016/S2215-0366(22)00161-4.

"PMDD in Young Adults: Premenstrual Dysphoric Disorder Symptoms and Treatment." Newport Institute, April 16, 2023. https://www.newportinstitute.com/resources/mental-health/premenstrual-dysphoric-disorder.

Polito, Vince. "Is Microdosing Just Placebo?" *Bill of Health* (blog). Petrie-Flom Center. Harvard Law School, April 7, 2022. https://blog.petrieflom.law.harvard.edu/2022/04/07/is-microdosing-just-placebo.

Polito, Vince, and Richard J. Stevenson. "A Systematic Study of Microdosing Psychedelics." *PLoS ONE* 14, no. 2 (February 2019): e0211023. https://doi.org/10.1371/journal.pone.0211023.

"Premenstrual Syndrome (PMS)." American College of Obstetricians and Gynecologists, November 2023. https://www.acog.org/womens-health/faqs/premenstrual-syndrome.

"Psilocybin and Epilepsy." Sanctuary Wellness Institute. https://sanctuarywellnessinstitute.com/psilocybin/psilocybin-and-epilepsy.php.

"Psilocybin and LSD in the Treatment of Cluster Headache." Clusterbusters, April 25, 2023. https://clusterbusters.org/resource/psilocybin-and-lsd-treatment.

"Psilocybin Mushrooms ('Magic Mushrooms')." Mother to Baby. Organization of Teratology Information Specialists (OTIS), May 2023. https://www.ncbi.nlm.nih.gov/books/NBK582810.

Puckett, Shae. "Psychedelics, the Microbiome, and IBD: A Next-Generation IBD Medication?" IBDCoach. https://ibd.coach/next-generation-drug.

r/Microdosing. Reddit. https://www.reddit.com/r/microdosing.

r/PsychedelicWomen. Reddit. https://www.reddit.com/r/PsychedelicWomen.

Rabin, Dave. "Feeling Safe Is the Key to Learning." Commune. Uploaded June 21, 2023. YouTube video, 1:00. https://www.youtube.com/watch?v=X7LB6fW_S1U.

Ramaekers, Johannes G., Nadia Hutten, Natasha L. Mason, Patrick Dolder, Eef L. Theunissen, Friederike Holze, Matthias E. Liechti, Amanda Feilding, and Kim P. C. Kuypers. "A Low Dose of Lysergic Acid Diethylamide Decreases Pain Perception in Healthy Volunteers." *Journal of Psychopharmacology* 35, no. 4 (April 2021): 398–405. https://doi.org/10.1177/0269881120940937.

Ravn, Pernille, Erik L. Secher, Ulrik Skram, Trine Therkildsen, Lona L. Christrup, and Mads U. Werner. "Morphine- and Buprenorphine-Induced Analgesia and Antihyperalgesia in a Human Inflammatory Pain Model: A Double-Blind, Randomized, Placebo-Controlled, Five-Arm Crossover Study." *Journal of Pain Research* 6 (January 2013): 23–38. https://doi.org/10.2147/JPR.S36827.

Raz, Shlomi. "Transforming Psychedelics into Mainstream Medicines." Stat. Boston Globe Media, January 7, 2020. https://www.statnews.com/2020/01/07/transforming-psychedelics-into-mainstream-medicines.

Resmovits, Joy. "ADHD Is Now Classified as a Specific Disability Under Federal Civil Rights Law." *Los Angeles Times,* July 26, 2016. https://latimes.com/local/education/la-na-adhd-disability-us-department-of-education-20160725-snap-story.html.

Roberts, Catherine. "How to Keep Ticks from Biting." *Consumer Reports,* April 21, 2023. https://www.consumerreports.org/health/outdoor-safety/how-to-keep-ticks-from-biting-a1206907538.

Romaszkan, Maria. "ADHD and Premenstrual Dysphoric Disorder." ADHD Online. Mentavi Health, April 17, 2023. https://adhdonline.com/articles/adhd-and-premenstrual-dysphoric-disorder.

Rootman, Joseph. "Findings from the Microdose.me Study: A Large Scale Observational Study of Psychedelic Microdosing." *Bill of Health* (blog). Petrie-Flom Center. Harvard Law School, April 14, 2022. https://blog.petrieflom.law.harvard.edu/2022/04/14/microdose-study.

Rootman, Joseph M., Maggie Kiraga, Pamela Kryskow, Kalin Harvey, Paul Stamets, Eesmyal Santos-Brault, Kim P. C. Kuypers, and Zach Walsh. "Psilocybin Microdosers Demonstrate Greater Observed Improvements in Mood and Mental Health at One Month Relative to Non-microdosing Controls." *Scientific Reports* 12, no. 1 (June 2022): 11091. https://doi.org/10.1038/s41598-022-14512-3.

Rootman, Joseph M., Pamela Kryskow, Kalin Harvey, Paul Stamets, Eesmyal Santos-Brault, Kim P. C. Kuypers, Vince Polito, Francoise Bourzat, and Zach Walsh. "Adults Who Microdose Psychedelics Report Health Related Motivations and Lower Levels of Anxiety and Depression Compared to Non-microdosers." *Scientific Reports–Nature* 11, no. 1 (November 2021): 22479. https://doi.org/10.1038/s41598-021-01811-4.

Rosenberg, Evan C., Richard W. Tsien, Benjamin J. Whalley, and Orrin Devinsky. "Cannabinoids and Epilepsy." *Neurotherapeutics* 12, no. 4 (October 2015): 747–68. https://doi.org/10.1007/s13311-015-0375-5.

Rouaud, Antonin, Abigail E. Calder, and Gregor Hasler. "Microdosing Psychedelics and the Risk of Cardiac Fibrosis and Valvulopathy: Comparison to Known Cardiotoxins." *Journal of Psychopharmacology*. Published ahead of print, January 12, 2024. https://doi.org/10.1177/02698811231225609.

Rudy, Lisa Jo. "What Does 'Neurotypical' Mean?" Verywell Health. Dotdash Meredith, August 08, 2023. https://www.verywellhealth.com/what-does-it-mean-to-be-neurotypical-260047.

Sanders, Laura. "A Chemical Imbalance Doesn't Explain Depression. So What Does?" *Science News,* February 12, 2023. https://www.sciencenews.org/article/chemical-imbalance-explain-depression.

Sansone, Randy A., and Lori A. Sansone. "SSRI-Induced Indifference." *Psychiatry* (Edgemont) 7, no. 10 (October 2010): 14–18.

Schindler, Emmanuelle A. D., R. Andrew Sewell, Christopher H. Gottschalk, Christina Luddy, L. Taylor Flynn, Hayley Lindsey, Brian P. Pittman, Nicholas V. Cozzi, and Deepak C. D'Souza. "Exploratory Controlled Study of the Migraine-Suppressing Effects of Psilocybin." *Neurotherapeutics* 18, no. 1 (January 2021): 534–43. https://doi.org/10.1007/s13311-020-00962-y.

Schmitt, Adolfo. "Incremental Calibration and Dosing Method Used by Microhuasca." Internal document, Microhuasca.

Shahar, Orr, Alexander Botvinnik, Amit Shwartz, Elad Lerer, Peretz Golding, Alex Buko,

Ethan Hamid, et al. "Effect of Chemically Synthesized Psilocybin and Psychedelic Mushroom Extract on Molecular and Metabolic Profiles in Mouse Brain." *Molecular Psychiatry*. Published ahead of print, February 20, 2024. https://doi.org/10.1038/s41380-024-02477-w.

Sharp, Jon, and Valerie Bonnelle. "Tiny Doses, Big Samples: The Largest Microdosing Study to Date." Beckley Foundation, November 29, 2021. https://www.beckleyfoundation.org/2021/11/29/tiny-doses-big-samples-the-largest-microdosing-study-to-date.

Sherman, Rachel E., Steven A. Anderson, Gerald J. Dal Pan, Gerry W. Gray, Thomas Gross, Nina L. Hunter, Lisa LaVange, et al. "Real-World Evidence—What Is It and What Can It Tell Us?" *New England Journal of Medicine* 375, no. 23 (December 2016): 2293–97. https://doi.org/10.1056/NEJMsb1609216.

Shoef, Wendy Perkins, Neuro-pleasure and ADHD coach, www.thesuccessdoula.com.

Siegel, Joshua S., Subha Subramanian, Demetrius Perry, Benjamin P. Kay, Evan M. Gordon, Timothy O. Laumann, T. Rick Reneau, et al. "Psilocybin Desynchronizes the Human Brain." *Nature* (July 2024). https://doi.org/10.1038/s41586-024-07624-5.

Sibley, Margaret H., Stephen V. Faraone, Joel T. Nigg, and Craig B. H. Surman. "Sudden Increases in U.S. Stimulant Prescribing: Alarming or Not?" *Journal of Attention Disorders* 27, no. 6 (April 2023): 571–74. https://doi.org/10.1177/10870547231164155.

Smith, Dana G. "Psychedelics Are a Promising Therapy, but They Can Be Dangerous for Some." *New York Times*, February 10, 2023. https://www.nytimes.com/2023/02/10/well/mind/psychedelics-therapy-ketamine-mushrooms-risks.html.

Sohn, Emily. "What Is 'Inflammaging'? Here's How Inflammation Affects You Differently as You Age." *National Geographic*, December 27, 2023. https://www.nationalgeographic.com/premium/article/inflammation-ache-pain-aging.

Solon, Olivia. "Under Pressure, Silicon Valley Workers Turn to LSD Microdosing." *Wired*, August 24, 2016. https://www.wired.co.uk/article/lsd-microdosing-drugs-silicon-valley.

Spotswood, C. J. *The Microdosing Guidebook*. Berkeley, CA: Ulysses Press, 2022.

Stafford, Peter, and Bonnie Golightly. "Education and the Psychedelics." Chap. 5 in *LSD: The Problem-Solving Psychedelic*. New York: Award Books, 1967. https://www.druglibrary.org/schaffer/lsd/staf5.htm.

Stamets, Paul. "How Paul Stamets STOPPED Stuttering | Joe Rogan Experience." Interview by Joe Rogan. JRE Archive. Uploaded February 15, 2023. YouTube video, 7:38. https://www.youtube.com/watch?v=ZEwKGUkW_ac.

Stannard, David E. *American Holocaust: The Conquest of the New World*. rev. ed. New York: Oxford University Press, 1993.

Stevenson, Shawn. *Sleep Smarter: 21 Essential Strategies to Sleep Your Way to a Better Body, Better Health, and Bigger Success*. New York: Rodale, 2016.

"Stuttering." National Institute on Deafness and Other Communication Disorders. US

Department of Health and Human Services, March 6, 2017. https://www.nidcd.nih .gov/health/stuttering.

Stuyt, Elizabeth. "The Problem with the Current High Potency THC Marijuana from the Perspective of an Addiction Psychiatrist." *Missouri Medicine* 115, no. 6 (November–December 2018): 482–86.

Suárez, Camila, Santiago Quintero, and Juan Miguel Cardona Gil. "Tendencias y experiencias del consumo de microdosis de hongos psilocibios en Colombia." *Cultura y Droga* 28, no. 35 (January 2023): 137–67. https://doi.org/10.17151/culdr.2023.28 .35.7.

"Summary Report (as of 2/26/2024)." NFL Concussion Settlement. https://www .nflconcussionsettlement.com/Reports_Statistics.aspx.

Szaflarski, Jerzy P., Elizabeth Martina Bebin, Anne M. Comi, Anup D. Patel, Charuta Joshi, Daniel Checketts, Jules C. Beal, et al. "Long-Term Safety and Treatment Effects of Cannabidiol in Children and Adults with Treatment-Resistant Epilepsies: Expanded Access Program Results." *Epilepsia* 59, no. 8 (August 2018): 1540–48. https://doi.org /10.1111/epi.14477.

Szigeti, Balázs, Laura Kartner, Allan Blemings, Fernando Rosas, Amanda Feilding, David J. Nutt, Robin L. Carhart-Harris, and David Erritzoe. "Self-Blinding Citizen Science to Explore Psychedelic Microdosing." *eLife* 10 (March 2021): e62878. https://doi.org /10.7554/eLife.62878.

Thiele, Elizabeth A., Eric D. Marsh, Jacqueline A. French, Maria Mazurkiewicz-Beldzinska, Selim R. Benbadis, Charuta Joshi, Paul D. Lyons, Adam Taylor, Claire Roberts, and Kenneth Sommerville. "Cannabidiol in Patients with Seizures Associated with Lennox-Gastaut Syndrome (GWPCARE4): A Randomised, Double-Blind, Placebo-Controlled Phase 3 Trial." *Lancet* 391, no. 10125 (March 2018): 1085–96. https://doi.org/10.1016/S0140-6736(18)30136-3.

Thomas, Kelan. "Safety First: Potential Heart Health Risks of Microdosing." *Bill of Health* (blog). Petrie-Flom Center. Harvard Law School, April 13, 2022. https://blog .petrieflom.law.harvard.edu/2022/04/13/safety-first-potential-heart-health-risks-of -microdosing.

Thompson, Caitlin, and Attila Szabo. "Psychedelics as a Novel Approach to Treating Autoimmune Conditions." *Immunology Letters* 228 (December 2020): 45–54. https:// doi.org/10.1016/j.imlet.2020.10.001.

Tiranini, Lara, and Rossella E. Nappi. "Recent Advances in Understanding/Management of Premenstrual Dysphoric Disorder/Premenstrual Syndrome." *Faculty Reviews* 11 (April 2022): 11. https://doi.org/10.12703/r/11-11.

"Traumatic Brain Injury." Johns Hopkins Medicine. https://www.hopkinsmedicine.org /health/conditions-and-diseases/traumatic-brain-injury.

Turner, Nicholas, dir. *Reimagining Prison* (webumentary). Vera Institute of Justice, October 2018. https://www.vera.org/reimagining-prison-webumentary.

u/Connect_Swim_8128. "Microdosing for bipolar 2/ADHD." r/Microdosing. Reddit, March 14, 2023. https://www.reddit.com/r/microdosing/comments/11r5dxm/microdosing_for_bipolar_2adhd.

u/jdyf333. "jdyf333: Overview." Reddit. https://www.reddit.com/user/jdyf333.

u/KaFaraqGatri07. "What's better for language learning: psilocybin, LSD, or DMT?" r/Microdosing. Reddit, March 26, 2019. https://www.reddit.com/r/microdosing/comments/b5qoxv/whats_better_for_language_learning_psilocybin_lsd.

u/lolfuys. "Scientists are beginning to unravel the effects of psilocybin mushrooms on bipolar disorder." r/Science. Reddit, January 21, 2023. https://www.reddit.com/r/science/comments/10i3vyg/scientists_are_beginning_to_unravel_the_effects. The account that originated this thread has since been suspended.

u/man_bear_pig_2. "Microdosing for sports performance, my experience." r/Microdosing. Reddit, July 13, 2021. https://www.reddit.com/r/microdosing/comments/ojrlhg/microdosing_for_sports_performance_my_experience.

u/nubpod23. "LSD or psilocybin microdosing good for stroke recovery?" r/Microdosing. Reddit, March 14, 2022. https://www.reddit.com/r/microdosing/comments/tdwkhr/lsd_or_psilocybin_microdosing_good_for_stroke.

u/Ok_Elevator6365. "Microdosing journey ends with Psychosis." r/Microdosing. Reddit, February 2, 2024. https://www.reddit.com/r/microdosing/comments/1ahaiag/microdose_journey_ended_with_psychosis.

u/SteRoPo. "Psilocybin microdosers demonstrate greater observed improvements in mood and mental health at one month relative to non-microdosing controls." r/Science. Reddit, June 30, 2022. https://www.reddit.com/r/science/comments/voepqy/psilocybin_microdosers_demonstrate_greater.

u/Vintagecrawfish. "Psilocybin stroke recovery." r/PsilocybinTherapy. Reddit, August 18, 2023. https://www.reddit.com/r/PsilocybinTherapy/comments/15umpjo/psilocybin_stroke_recovery.

Ulrich, Austin. "10 Possible Side Effects of Combination Inhalers." GoodRX Health, June 24, 2022. https://www.goodrx.com/drugs/side-effects/10-common-side-effects-of-combination-inhalers.

Van de Plassche, Peggy. "Psychedelic Productivity: Can Microdosing Psilocybin Boost Your Performance at Work?" Interview by Briana Supardi. CBS6 Albany. Sinclair, December 5, 2023. https://cbs6albany.com/news/local/psychedelic-productivity-can-microdosing-psilocybin-boost-your-performance-at-work-magic-mushrooms-van-de-plassche-medicine-drugs.

Vandergriendt, Carly. "All About Persistent Postural-Perceptual Dizziness (PPPD)." Healthline, April 19, 2023. https://www.healthline.com/health/persistent-postural-perceptual-dizziness#outlook.

Wade, Grace. "Microdosing LSD Increases the Complexity of Your Brain Signals." *New Scientist*, February 15, 2024. https://www.newscientist.com/article/2416478-microdosing-lsd-increases-the-complexity-of-your-brain-signals.

Waldman, Ayelet. *A Really Good Day: How Microdosing Made a Mega Difference in My Mood, My Marriage, and My Life.* New York: Knopf, 2017.

Watson, D., L. A. Clark, and A. Tellegen. "Development and Validation of Brief Measures of Positive and Negative Affect: The PANAS Scales." *Journal of Personality and Social Psychology* 54, no. 6 (June 1988): 1063–70. https://doi.org/10.1037/0022-3514.54.6.1063.

Week Staff. "ADHD: The Trouble with Diagnosis." *The Week,* May 17, 2023. https://theweek.com/news/science-health/960875/adhd-the-trouble-with-diagnosis.

Weisberg, D. M. *Cannabis Roadmap: Medical Marijuana Guide for Optimal Health and Wellness.* Self-published, Amazon Digital Services, 2023.

"What Is ADHD?" Centers for Disease Control and Prevention. US Department of Health and Human Services, September 27, 2023. https://www.cdc.gov/ncbddd/adhd/facts.html.

"What Is Cerebral Palsy?" Centers for Disease Control and Prevention. US Department of Health and Human Services, February 28, 2024. https://www.cdc.gov/ncbddd/cp/facts.html.

"What Is Eczema?" National Eczema Association. https://nationaleczema.org/eczema.

"What Is Persistent Postural Perceptual Dizziness (PPPD)?" Ménière's Society. https://www.menieres.org.uk/information-and-support/symptoms-and-conditions/pppd.

Wietstock, Cara. "Lemon Tek: The Citrus-Based Magic Mushroom Hack." GreenState. Hearst Communications, September 8, 2023. https://www.greenstate.com/explained/lemon-tek-magic-mushroom-hack.

Wilber, Ken. *The Many Ways We Touch: Three Principles Helpful for Any Integrative Approach.* Self-published, Integral Life, 2006. https://integral-life-home.s3.amazonaws.com/Wilber-TheManyWaysWeTouch.pdf.

Wilcox, Anna. "Microdosing LSA: People Are Microdosing Acid's Less Known, Legal Cousin." *DoubleBlind,* February 24, 2021. https://doubleblindmag.com/microdosing-lsa-morning-glory-seeds.

Williams, Tina. "Hailey's Microdosing Journey." *Menstrual Moods and Mushrooms* (blog). Substack, April 21, 2023. https://tinawill.substack.com/p/haileys-microdosing-journey.

Zarankin, Mariana, Maria S. Pellegrini, and Francisco Zenteno. "Psilocybin Fungi Microdose Treatment in Major Depressive Disorder: A Case Report." [In Spanish.] *Vertex Revista Argentina De Psiquiatría* 35, no. 164 (April–June 2024): 33–39. https://doi.org/10.53680/vertex.v35i164.544.

Index

academics, improved grades and, 91–92

Adam. *See* MDMA

ADD. *See* attention deficit disorder

Adderall, 109, 111–13

addiction, 10, 201–2

ADHD. *See* attention deficit/hyperactivity disorder

ALD-52, 28

Algernon Pharmaceuticals, 219

All Things Amanita website, 59

allergic asthma, 164

Alpert, Richard. *See* Dass, Ram

Amanita muscaria (mushroom type), 29, 37, 38, 61

   legal status of, 49, 72

   location found, 49

   Masha book on, 168, 197

   microdosing with, 48–50

   preparation process, 49

   protocols, 59–60

   sleep protocol for, 215

   substance verification and, 57

American Psychiatric Association, 129–30

amphetamines, 115–16

anorexia (anorexia nervosa), 159–62

antidepressants, 43, 65, 93

   classified, 121–22

   different effects of microdosing and, 126–28

   federal studies of long-term use of, 71

   negative reports on, 122

   psilocybin microdose *vs.*, 161

   serotonin theory and, 129–31

"Anti-inflammatory Therapeutics" (Nichols), 259

anxiety, 52, 112, 162, 163, 164

application program interface (API), 97

ASD. *See* autism spectrum disorder

Asperger's. *See* autism

aspirin, 65, 75

asthma, 164–66, 259

The Atlantic, 253

attention deficit disorder (ADD), 114, 116

attention deficit/hyperactivity disorder (ADHD), 92, 108

   Adderall alternative and, 109, 111–13

attention deficit (*continued*)
amphetamines access and, 115–16
benefits duration, 118–20
in children, 116–18
diagnosis difficulty of, 115
evening dosing and, 113
medications, 120–21
neuroplasticity windows and, 255–56
parental pressure for continuing
medications, 116
personal reports on, 110–14
research reports on, 114
rise in diagnosed cases of, 115
when effects of microdosing are felt,
114
Autism on Acid (Orsini), 168
autism spectrum disorder (ASD)
children and severe, 169–71
high functioning (Asperger's),
166–69
neurodivergence and, 167
ayahuasca, 28, 38, 48, 250
children and, 84
indigenous use of, 145
mixture and procedure for making,
47
Aztecs, 40

Beckley Foundation, 228, 229–31
benefits, 13. *See also* health conditions;
wellness, enhanced abilities and;
specific health conditions
general, 3
parenting, 151–52
side, 186, 187
two categories of, 14–15
unexpected, 202, *243*
best practices
integration, 79
minimum duration, 80
mixing high and low doses, 74–75
recommendations for coaches, retreats,
groups, 78
regular day, 79–80
set and setting, 78–79
sourcing psychedelics, 72–74
trauma-informed practitioner and,
76–77
working with others, 80–81
Bezos, Jeff, 288
binge eating, 171–72
bipolar disorder, 172–74
Blotter (Davis), 39
body weight, 53, 174
Bramlage, Adam (coach), 184
Breaking Convention conference, 211
Burning Man, 69

cacao, 40
Canadian Phase 2A clinical trial, 132
cannabis (marijuana), 28–30, 36
reducing or quitting, 175–76
Carcillo, Daniel, 223
cerebral palsy (CP), 176–78
ceremonial cacao, 40
chickenpox, 224
childbirth, early, 109
children
ADHD in, 116–18
ayahuasca given to, 84
eczema in, 183
severe autism and, 169–71
Chinese medicine, stacking and, 41
chocolate, 101–2
chronic pain, 139–41
Church of Ambrosia, 282
citizen science, 236, 237–38,
276–77
Clearlight Brand, 270, 271
Clinton, Hillary, 7
cluster headaches, 179–80, 198
Clusterbusters.org, 179–80

coaches and coaching
    eczema testimonial from, 184
    integration and, 79
    on microdosing for ADHD, 119
    "microdosing professionals" and,
        280–81
    questions to ask potential, 80–81
    recommendations for, 78
    TBI client example, 41
    trauma-informed, 76–77
    use of term, 25
    working with "friend group" instead
        of, 81
coding, math and, 97–98
cognition, enhanced, 87–88
color blindness, 180–81
common cold, 181–82
community, microdosing, 6–7, 16
concerns and controversies, 16–18
contraindications, 25
    medications and conditions, 70
    psychotic episodes, 67–68
    side effects and, 64–67
    taking too much by mistake, 68–70
CP. *See* cerebral palsy
creativity, 88–89, 113
Crohn's disease, 190
Csikszentmihalyi, Mihaly, 90
cultural appropriation, 265, 267–69
"The Curious Connection Between
    Psychedelics and Longevity"
    (Haigney), 96
cytokines, 258

Dass, Ram (Richard Alpert), 235
DASS-21 scale, 229
Davis, Erik, 39
Davy, Humphry, 234–35
DEA. *See* Drug Enforcement
    Administration
decarboxylation, 49

default mode network (DMN), 253–56
defense, repair, and maintenance (DRM),
    96
Delos Psyche Research Group, 204–5
dementia, 281
depression, 108, 112
    alleviation of severe, 113
    anxiety associated with, 163
    benefits for, 124–28
    fatigue factor in, 131
    first study designed for microdosing
        and, 128–29
    general information about, 121–24
    high-dose psychedelics for, 122
    lack of knowledge about, 129
    long-term, 93–94
    measuring, 129
    reason for microdosing improving, 132
    serotonin theory of, 129–31
Diamond Shruumz–Brand products, 12
distance running, 104–5
dizziness. *See* persistent postural
    perceptual dizziness
DMN. *See* default mode network
DMT. *See* N,N-dimethyltryptamine
doctors, 24–25
The Doors of Perception (Huxley), 235
dosage, 18, 33, 201. *See also specific
    conditions; specific substances*
    body weight and, 53
    convenient psilocybin tabs and, 74
    decreasing, 53–54
    depression study and, 128
    desire to increase, 54–55
    eliminating negative effects through, 65
    experimenting with, 54
    how recommendations arose for, 44–45
    individual and specific situation as
        criteria for, 82
    mixing high and low, 74–75
    optimal dose level changes, 50–51

dosage (*continued*)
   for other substances, 46–50
   overdose potential, 55–57
   psychedelic effects level and, 44
   radically higher, 52–53
   radically smaller, 51–52
   taking too much by mistake, 68–70
   variability, 53–54
   verifying substance and, 57–58
   when to lower, 51
dot-com boom, 107
double-blind method, 233, 288
drinking, 187
DRM. *See* defense, repair, and maintenance
Drug Enforcement Administration
      (DEA), 35–36, 73
DysphoricProject.org, 211

Earth Wisdom archive. *See* Erowid
eating disorders, 171. *See also* binge eating
ecstasy. *See* MDMA
eczema, 183–84
Ehlers-Danlos syndrome (EDS), 184–88,
      258
elixirs, 282
Ellis, Dock, 102
emotions, daily checklist of, 92–93
enhanced abilities. *See* wellness, enhanced
      abilities and
enhanced cognition, 87–88
epilepsy, 188–89
Erowid (Earth Wisdom), 84
Eubanks, Chris, 94–95
Exeter, England, 232–33
expectations, 21, 239, 241–43
   benefits beyond, 202, *243*

Facebook, bipolar group on, 173
Fadiman, Jim, 6, 54, 73, 75, 273, 288–89
   new chapter by, 283
   protocol, 59, 60, 61

father of modern microdosing, 5
FDA. *See* Food and Drug Administration
Feilding, Amanda, 284
Ferriss, Tim, 87–88, 273
Fireside Project hotline, 10
Fisher, Gary, 170–71
5-HT(2A), 165, 257
flow, concept of, 90
Fly Agaric (Feeney), 48–49. *See also*
      Amanita muscaria
focus, increased ability to, 89–90, 95
Food and Drug Administration (FDA),
      12, 32, 233
food choices, better, 90–91
Forbes, 274
Forte, Robert, 44, 272
Fried, Eiko, 129
Friedman, Richard A., 253–54
friend group, 81

Gaia, 286
gender, stuttering and, 219
"Get-More-Out-Of-This-Life" kit, 26
grades, academics and, 91–92
greed, 278–80
Griffiths, Roland, 61
groups, microdosing, 78
Gruber, Jordan, 6, 54
The Guardian, 96
gummies, 74

Haden, Mark, 213–14
Hahnemann, Samuel, 262
Haigney, Zach, 96
hallucinations, 19, 212
Hamilton Depression Scale, 128
happiness, 161
Harvard Group, 1960s, 268
Hashkes, Sarah, 240
Hasler, 248–49, 251
Hawaiian baby woodrose seeds, 37, 50

headaches
   cluster, 109,179–80
   migraine, 189–90, 198
health conditions
   heart damage concerns and, 260–61
   information sources, 81–83
   minors and, 84
   not covered, 3–4
   physical, 14
   research and, 25–26
   single case extrapolation, 83–84
   symptoms benefited and, 81–83
   2060 vision and, 289
health conditions, positively affected. *See also* wellness, enhanced abilities and; women's health
   anorexia, 159–62
   anxiety, 162–64
   asthma, 164–66
   autism, 166–71
   binge eating, 171–72
   bipolar disorder, 172–74
   body weight, 174
   cerebral palsy case study, 176–78
   cluster headaches, 179–80, 198
   color blindness (red-green), 180–81
   common cold, 181–82
   commonalities and generalizations, 157–59
   dizziness (PPPD) case study, 182–83
   eczema, 183–84
   Ehlers-Danlos syndrome (EDS), 184–88
   epilepsy, 188–89
   inflammation, 256–60
   inflammatory bowel disease (IBD), 190–91
   libido lacking, 191
   lupus case study, 192–93
   Lyme disease, 193–97
   migraine headaches, 189–90, 198

   multiple sclerosis (MS), 197–200
   palliative care and, 200–201
   post-traumatic stress disorder (PTSD), 203–5
   premenstrual dysphoric disorder (PMDD), 206–11
   premenstrual syndrome (PMS), 211–12
   schizophrenia, 212–14
   sleep and, 214–16
   stroke, 216–19
   stuttering, 219–21
   traumatic brain injury (TBI), 221–23
   varicella-zoster virus (shingles), 224–26
heart damage, concerns over, 260–61
herbal mixtures, 101–2
hesitation, value of, 22–23
hockey player, report on pain alleviation, 142
Hofmann, Albert, 31–32, 235
   dosage taken by, 44
   Wasson and, 266
homeopathy, 262–63
Hooke, Robert, 234
hotline, 10
"How Psilocybin Can Rewire Our Brain" (podcast episode), 255
HPOTS. *See* hyperadrenergic postural orthostatic tachycardia syndrome
Huberman, Andrew, 255
human potential, 286–89
Huxley, Aldous, 75, 235, 286
hyperadrenergic postural orthostatic tachycardia syndrome (HPOTS), 137

IBD. *See* inflammatory bowel disease
ibogaine, 28
ibuprofen, 75
illegal substances, in US, 28, 32, 35–36
Imperial College, 228

indigenous people
  ayahuasca use by, 145
  blending indigenous and Western use,
    269
  consciousness-altering substances, use
    by, 40
  cultural appropriation question and,
    265, 267–69
  medicines and ethical principles, 266
  microdosing development independent
    of, 267–69
  psychedelics viewed by, 283
inflammation, 256–59
inflammatory bowel disease (IBD),
    190–91, 259
Institute of Noetic Sciences, 277
integration, 79
intranasal sprays, 29
Intuitive Protocol, 59, 60

Jesus, Sufi story about, 69–70
Jewell, Tim, 167
Johns Hopkins University, 61
jujitsu, 102–3

ketamine, 29, 161
kickboxing, 104
Kinderlehrer, Daniel, 196
Knowles, Richard, 204
Korb, Jim, 88, 92
Korb, Sophia, 37, 88, 92
  data collection idea of, 273
  shingles relief and, 224–25

language learning, 94–95
Latifi, Fortesa, 101
Leary, Tim, 235, 268, 286
legality, 21, 33, 73, 150. *See also specific
    substances*
  enforcement and, 72
  legalization benefits and, 58

as location dependent, 23
  minors and, 84
  politics of, 35–36, 37, 72
  Schedule I drugs and, 35–36
lemon-tekking, 41, 42–43
libido, 99, 113, 191
lion's mane mushroom, 40
liver, 51, 75
long COVID, 108, 259
  definition of term, 132–33
  reports, 133–37
longevity, 96
LSA-morning glory seeds, 28, 37, 50
LSD. *See* lysergic acid diethylamide
LSD-25, 31–32
lupus, 192–93
Lyme disease, 193–97
lysergic acid diethylamide (LSD), 28, 29,
    36, 270, 271
  availability of, 268
  black market for, 33
  cactus properties identical to, 37
  cannabis *vs.*, 30
  cells impacted by, 33
  chemist responsible for creating, 268
  clinical success in treating depression
    with, 132
  common microdose size, 33
  creator of, 31, 267
  dangerous substances sold as, 57
  dosage, 33, 44–45
  Hofmann experiments with, 31–32
  Leary first experience of, 268
  legal status of, 33
  long-term safety of, 71
  microdose method for, 38–39
  molecules, 33
  neural complexity increased by, 30
  optimum dose level for psilocybin and,
    45–46
  preferences for, 95

psilocybin compared to, 37–38, 177
Reddit post on, 95
as Schedule I drug, 36
shift to mushrooms from, 280
taking too much by mistake, 68–69
transcendent approach to taking, 5
Waldman account of sourcing, 73

macrodosing, 75, 286
magic mushrooms. *See* mushrooms;
 psilocybin
MALS. *See* median arcuate ligament
 syndrome
manic-depressive disorder. *See* bipolar
 disorder
MAPS. *See* Multidisciplinary Association
 for Psychedelic Studies
marijuana. *See* cannabis
Masha, Baba, 168, 188–89, 197, 219
 protocol, 59
Maslow, Abraham, 233
math, coding and, 97–98
Mayo Clinic, 171
McKenna, Dennis, 104
MD. *See* microdosing and microdoses
MDMA ("Ecstasy"), 29, 36, 203, 205, 260
ME/CFS. *See* myalgic encephalomyelitis/
 chronic fatigue syndrome
median arcuate ligament syndrome
 (MALS), 135
medical marijuana, 30
medications, 85, 120–21, 187
 blending microdosing and, 112–13
 parental support for keeping students
  on, 116
 reflexive reach-back, 119
 tapering off, 108, 137–39
Medium.com, 94–95
menopause, 208, 209
mental health, 21, 26
 Beckley report measure of, 229–31

benefits, 14
longevity and, 96
mescaline, 8, 31, 36, 71
Microdose.me Survey, 228–31
microdosing and microdoses, 1–4. *See also*
 dosage; modern microdosing; *specific*
 topics
amount, 18
anti-addictive nature of, 10
blending medications with, 112–13
breastfeeding while, 147–50
combinations and, 39–40
community, 6–7, 16
concerns and controversies, 16–18
contraindications, 70
cumulative effects of, 62
daily, 62–63
finding substances for, 24
first extensive study on, 29
first use of term, 270–72
first-time, 60
gathering reports on, 5
homeopathy compared to, 262–63
human potential and, 286–89
macrodosing *vs.*, 286
meaning of, 8, 9, 30
method of taking, 38–39
minimum duration for, 80
by mistake, 10
misuse of word, 11–12, 29–30
motivation for, 21
onset of effects, 43–44
overlooked, 32
popularity, 15–16, 276
protocols (schedules), 58–61
psychotherapy and, 77
psychotic episodes and, 67–68
real-life evidence, 277
reasons for not, 20–22
regular day and, 79–80
reports from people who stopped, 22

microdosing and microdoses (*continued*)
  research review on effects of, 20
  safety, 9–12, 16–17, 51, 70–71
  second-day effect of, 61
  side effects of, 64–67
  social, 100–102
  stimulant *vs.* general system enhancer
    view of, 214–15
  studies, 13
  "sub-perceptual" description of, 18–20
  substances not recommended for, 29
  substances used for, 28–31
  takeaways, 287–89
  taking only one, 61–62
  time off from, 60, 63–64
  uncomfortable effects from, 65–67
  underground test lab, 11
  vitamins and, 71
  website, 182
  well-being and, 26
  why people try, 12–13
Microdosing Institute of the Netherlands,
    215, 222
Microdosing Institute Protocol, 59
Microdosing with Amanita Muscaria
    (Masha), 168, 197
MicrodosingPsychedelics.com, 92
Microhausca group, in Peru, 269
migraine headaches, 189–90, 198
MIND VITAMIN TABLETS, 270, 271
MindBio Therapeutics, 132
mindset. *See* set and setting
minors, 84
MMA, 103
modern microdosing, 4, 30–31, 227, 236
  beginning of, 272–74
"more-mores," 54
morning glory seeds. *See* LSA-morning
    glory seeds
Mothers of the Mushroom Project, 144
MS. *See* multiple sclerosis

Multidisciplinary Association for
    Psychedelic Studies (MAPS), 203–4,
    222–23
  Haden report on schizophrenia,
    213–14
multiple sclerosis (MS), 197, 198–200
mushrooms, 22, 28, 144. *See also Amanita
    muscaria;* psilocybin
  combinations of cacao and sacred, 40
  cultivars, 263
  jujitsu practitioner on, 102–3
  legal status of, 72–73
  low cost and variety of, 280
  new products and, 282
  new underground products of, 282
  number of psilocybin-containing, 263
  personal accounts of depression relief
    through microdosing with, 124–26
  presence or "being" experiences with,
    38
  psilocybin-containing, 39
  shift from LSD to, 280
  surprises from microdosing with,
    153–54
musicians, 98
Myco, Mikaela de la, 144, 145
myalgic encephalomyelitis/chronic fatigue
    syndrome (ME/CFS), 137

Nader, Ralph, 286
National Association of Anorexia Nervosa
    and Associated Disorders, 159–60
National Eczema Association, 183
National Football League, 222
National Institutes of Health, 171, 219,
    228, 263
National Institute of Mental Health, 173
neurodivergence, 167
neuroplasticity, 199, 258
  default mode network (DMN) and,
    253–56

mushrooms and, 264
neurogenesis and, 244–48
therapeutic and negative, 252–53
windows, 254, 255–56
New England Journal of Medicine, 131
The New York Times, 68
The New Yorker, 282
Nichols, Charles, 259
nightcap protocol, 59, 60, 215
Nixon, Richard, 35–36
N,N-dimethyltryptamine (DMT), 28, 29, 71, 219
"nocebo," 239
Nutt, David, 157, 228, 241, 242

obsessive-compulsive disorder (OCD), 112
opiates, federal regulations on, 141–42
Orsini, Aaron, 167–68
overdose, 55–57, 68–70

pain, 140, 144, 225
management, 108, 141–42
reports on help with, 141–43
statistics, 139
palliative care, 200–201
pandemic, 16
parenting, 151–53
parties, 100–102
Passie, Torsten, 270
Paxlovid, 137
persistent Lyme disease syndrome. *See* Lyme disease
persistent postural perceptual dizziness (PPPD), 182–83
Peru, Microhausca group in, 269
peyote, 28
pharmaceuticals, 32, 44, 70–71, 219
safety of microdosing *vs.,* 11
physical conditions. *See* health conditions

placebo effect, 18, 240–41. *See also* expectations
cartoon, *19*
controversy, 238–39
definition and usage, 239
expectations and, 21, 239
misapplied criteria and, 288
plane analogy, 277–78
PMDD. *See* premenstrual dysphoric disorder
PMS. *See* premenstrual syndrome
podcasts, 255, 273
Pollan, Michael, 75
popularity, 15–16, 276
pornography addiction, 201–2
post-traumatic stress disorder (PTSD), 203–5
PPPD. *See* persistent postural perceptual dizziness
predictions, 278–83
preexisting physical conditions, 20–21
pregnancy, 109, 145–47
premenstrual dysphoric disorder (PMDD), 206–11
premenstrual syndrome (PMS), 211–12
profit, greed and, 278–80
protocols, microdose, 58–61. *See also specific health conditions*
Psilocybe Mexicana, 43
psilocybin ("magic" mushrooms), 28, 29
antidepressants *vs.,* 161
decriminalization of, 34
ease of use, 74
home-grown cultivation of, 34
important facts about, 33–35
indigenous use and, 265, 267–69
laboratory-grown, 34
legal status of, 33–34
liver conversion of, 51
LSD compared with, 37–38, 177
microdosing form of, 34

psilocybin (*continued*)

mushrooms containing, 39

Nixon campaign against, 35–36

number of species, 33

optimum dose level for LSD and, 45–46

psychoactive properties, 34

QTest, 57

Sandoz-synthesized, 32, 268

spore print, 34

stacking with, 40–41

synthesized *vs.* extract, 263–65

The Psychedelic Explorer's Guide (Fadiman), 6, 73, 75, 273, 288–89

chapter added to, 283

predictions made in, 278

"Psychedelic Legalization & Decriminalization Tracker," 21

Psychedelic Science conference, MAPS, 203–4

psychedelics, 8, 210

addictive question, 10

afterglow from large dose, 254–55

availability of, 16

becoming illegal, 4

churches of, 281, 282

conference in Exeter on, 232–33

finding substances and, 24

future research on, 231

high-dose effects and, 75

legislation on, 35

LSD as basis of interest in, 268

microdose *vs.* full dose of, 18

other, non-"classic," 30–31

peer support line, 10

quality and purity of, 21–22

renaissance, 87

as safe, 65

safety and, 10

schizophrenic episodes from high-dose, 213

sourcing of, 72–74

"sub-perceptual" and, 18–20

as teachers, 283

psychiatric drugs, 1960s research and, 32

psychotherapy, 77

psychotic episodes, 67–68

PTSD. *See* post-traumatic stress disorder

PubMed, 228

qualifications of authors, 4–7

A Really Good Day (Waldman), 73, 274

Reddit, 16, 83, 173, 217

asthma relief testimonials on, 165

autism comments on, 168–69

LSD comment on, 95

post on increased focus, 95

"psychedelic women" thread on, 210

sex drive comment on, 98

red-green color blindness, 20–21

Refinery29, 101

regular day, 79–80

reports, microdosing, 228. *See also specific* conditions

Erowid.org vaults of, 37–38

formal research *vs.* personal, 234–37, 241

gathering and sharing experience, 285–86

gathering process, 5

LSD *vs.* psilocybin, 37–38

most prevalent substances in, 29

project surprises and challenges, 285–86

real-life evidence via, 277

research, 20, 204–5. *See also* science; *specific topics*

Canadian Phase 2A clinical trial, 132

on cannabis *vs.* LSD, 30

default mode network (DMN), 253–56

double-blind method of, 233, 288

funding, 228

future psychedelic, 231

"gold standard" for, 233

gradual increase in, 227–28

health conditions and, 25–26

individual experiences *vs.* formal, 283–84

issues, 275–76

LSD and 1970s, 36

microdosing survey of 80 countries, 40–41

on negative effects, 66

1960s psychiatric drug, 32

personal reports *vs.* formal, 234–37, 241

pharmaceutical studies and, 70–71

problem with experimental, 233

reason for lack of definitive, 228

sleep study, 100

"spontaneous healings" study, 277

substances available for, 33

website for cluster headaches, 179–80

wrong methodologies for studying microdosing, 233

research, current findings in, 228

ADHD, 114–21

chronic pain recent studies, 139–41

depression, 123–32

help with chronic pain, 139–45

long COVID reports, 133–37

mushroom journey surprises, 153–54

pain reports, 141–43

palliative care, 200–201

parenting, 151–53

tapering off medications, 108, 137–39

women's health, 108, 144–58

retreats, 78

Rogan, Joe, 104

Rolling Stone, 87, 274

Rootman, Joseph, 230

Rose, Davivid, 270–72

Royal College of London, 168

Royal Society of London, 231, 234–36

running, distance, 104–5

Sabina, María, 266–67, 269

safety, 9–12, 16–17, 70–71

lowering dose levels for, 51

Salvia divinorum, 29

San Francisco Psychedelic Society, 97

San Pedro cactus, 38, 57

legal status of LSD *vs.,* 36–37

Sanders, Laura, 131

Sanders, Nick, 268

Sandoz Pharmaceuticals, 32, 44

Schedule I drugs, 35–36

schedules. *See* protocols, microdose

schizophrenia, 212–14

science, 287. *See also* neuroplasticity

citizen, 236, 237–38, 276–77

contemporary observational, 231–37

expectations and, 202, 241–43, *243*

gradual increase in research, 227–28

history of, 231–32, 234–37

placebo effect and, 18, *19,* 238–41, 288

safety from perspective of, 17–18

scientific revolution and, 231–33

Scientific American, 68

Scientific Reports—Nature, 228

scopaesthesia, 102

second-day effect, 61

selective serotonin-reuptake inhibitors (SSRIs), 93, 121

downsides of, 130–31

PMDD and, 207, 208

serotonin hypothesis and, 129

tapering off, 138–39

serotonin, depression and, 129–31

set and setting, 78–79

sex drive. *See* libido

sexual enhancement, 98–99

shingles (varicella-zoster virus), 25–26,
    224–26
Shipibo-Conibo shamans, 145, 269
Shoef, Wendy Perkins, 119
side effects, 10, 66–67
    scam, 64–65
Silicon Valley, 87–88, 107, 273, 274
    CEOs with Asperger's, 167
sleep, 99–100, 186, 214–16
smoking, 187, 230
social anxiety, 52, 163
social issues, 275
social microdoses, 100–102
spiritual benefits, 14
sports and athletics, 102–5
SSRIs. *See* selective serotonin-reuptake
    inhibitors
stacking, 40, 41
Stamets, Paul, 40–41
    Stamets Protocol, 59, 60
    stuttering cure experience of, 219–21
stroke, 216–19
students, 97, 98, 104
    ADD/ADHD medication pressure on,
    116
stuttering, 219–21
"sub-perceptual," 18–20
substances, 27. *See also* psychedelics;
    specific substances
    cacao, 40
    beyond "classic" psychedelics, 30–31
    combinations of, 39–40
    comments on preferred, 95
    dosage for other, 46–50
    finding, 24
    illegal in US, 28, 32, 35–36
    interest in consciousness-altering, 269
    new and old, 280–81, 282
    not recommended for microdosing, 29
    research, 33
    stacking, 40

used for microdosing, 28–31
    verifying dosage and, 57–58
sub-threshold, 8, 19
Sufi tradition, Jesus story in, 69–70
suicidal thoughts, 153, 223
suicide headaches. *See* cluster headaches
support groups, 78. *See also* community,
    microdosing
    "friend groups" as, 81

tap test, 40–41
TBI. *See* traumatic brain injury
test kits, 57
THC, 30
therapists, need for experienced, 25
therapy
    MDMA-assisted, 203, 205
    trauma-informed, 76
TikTok, 73
The Times (London), 74
tinnitus, 20
Tolson, Naomi, 144
tracers, 20–21, 180
transformation, 284–85
traumas, 76–77
traumatic brain injury (TBI), 221–23
tune-up analogy, 88
Tylenol, 65

UC Berkeley, 73
United States (US)
    federal government, 71
    leading cause of adult death in, 216
    substances illegal in, 28, 32

vaccinations, 137
valvular heart disease (VHD), 260,
    261
vape pens, 29
varicella-zoster virus. *See* shingles
VHD. *See* valvular heart disease

"The Viability of Microdosing
    Psychedelics as a Strategy to
    Enhance Cognition and Well-being"
    (Bornemann, 2020), 86
vision improvement, 105–6
vitamins, 40, 71. *See also* MIND
    VITAMIN TABLETS
vodka, 39
volleyball, 104
Vyvanse, 113

Waldman, Ayelet, 73, 274
The Wall Street Journal, 74
Wasson, R. Gordon, 266
weddings, 101
wellness, enhanced abilities and
    benefits duration and, 120
    better food choices, 90–91
    creativity enhancement (art), 88–89
    enhanced cognition, 87–88
    flow and, 86–87
    grades and academics improvement,
        91–92
    happiness, 92–93
    increased ability to focus, 89–90, 95
    language learning, 94–95
    longevity, 96
    for musicians, 98
    sexual enhancement, 98–99
    sleep quality, 99–100

social microdoses and, 100–102
sports and athletics, 102–5
students on, 97–98
vision improvement, 105–6
work quality improvement, 107
Wired UK, 274
Wixarika (Huichol) group, 145
women, "psychedelic" (Reddit),
    210
women's health, 108, 109
    breastfeeding, 147–50
    overview, 144–45
    parenting benefits, 151–52
    parenting challenges, 152–53
    postpartum period, 149, 153–56
    pregnancy, 145–47
    recommendations, 155–56
    surprises on mushroom journey,
        153–54
    telling others about microdosing and,
        154–55
work quality improvement, 107
"Worldwide Psychedelic Laws Tracker,"
    21
writing, 89

Your Symphony of Selves (Fadiman/
    Gruber), 6, 54

Zendo Project, 69

About the Authors

James Fadiman, PhD, has been professionally involved with psychedelics for more than sixty years. He developed modern microdosing, including the use of protocols, specific dose ranges, and time off. The author of *The Psychedelic Explorer's Guide,* he has also written textbooks, professional books, a self-help book, a novel, and videos for PBS. He has taught at three universities, run his own management consulting firm, cofounded the Institute of Transpersonal Psychology, and served as the director of the Institute of Noetic Science.

Jordan Gruber, JD, coauthor of *Your Symphony of Selves* with Fadiman in 2020, has written, ghostwritten, and edited more than a dozen books in a wide variety of fields, from forensics and finances to fitness and psychology. In the mid-1990s, he founded the Enlightenment.com website. He has been close friends with Fadiman since 1990 and contributed to *The Psychedelic Explorer's Guide.*